The Gastrointestinal System at a Glance

The Gastrointestinal System at a Glance

SATISH KESHAV

MBBCh (Wits), DPhil (Oxon), MRCP (UK)
Consultant Gastroenterologist
Director, Centre for Gastroenterology
Royal Free and University College Medical School
University College London
Rowland Hill Street
London NW3 2PF

Blackwell
Science

First published 2004

Library of Congress Cataloging-in-Publication Data

Keshav, Satish.
    The gastrointestinal system at a glance/Satish Keshav. — 1st ed.
        p.   ;   cm.
Includes index.
ISBN 0-632-05472-7
    1. Gastrointestinal system.   2. Gastrointestinal system — Diseases.
    [DNLM: 1. Digestive System. 2. Digestive System Diseases. WI 100
    K42g 2003] I. Title.
    QP145.K447 2003
    612.3′2 — dc21
                            2003004942

ISBN 0-632-05472-7

A catalogue record for this title is available from the British Library

Set in 9/11.5 Times by SNP Best-set Typesetter Ltd., Hong Kong
Printed and bound in the United Kingdom by Ashford Colour Press, Gosport

Commissioning Editor: Fiona Goodgame
Managing Editor: Geraldine Jeffers
Production Editor: Fiona Pattison
Production Controller: Kate Charman

For further information on Blackwell Publishing, visit our website:
http://www.blackwellpublishing.com

Contents

Preface

How to use this book

This book presents a graphic scaffold for further detailed study and is an aid to revision. Therefore, it will be useful for students approaching a subject for the first time, particularly as part of an integrated systems-based medical curriculum. The diagrams will make abstract concepts more memorable and help the student to recall details that might otherwise be lost in plain text. The student may further annotate the diagrams with additional details from lectures, tutorials and self-directed study, to help with later revision.

Organization of the book

The book is organized in four parts, starting with a structural and functional overview of the main components of the gastrointestinal system, followed by consideration of integrated gastrointestinal function, which requires some preceding basic knowledge. Clinical examples are included throughout these early chapters highlighting the practical importance of each subject.

The third and fourth sections are more clinical, and cover the most important gastrointestinal and hepatobiliary diseases and the main aspects of diagnosis and treatment. Fundamental pathophysiological mechanisms are emphasized.

Anatomical and clinical detail

The anatomical diagrams are functional representations, and not exact reproductions, and they are used to illustrate how structure supports function.

Similarly, specific diseases are discussed to demonstrate pathogenic mechanisms and general principles, rather than to provide exhaustive detail. This book should be used to understand the normal physiology, how it goes wrong in disease, and the principles underlying modern clinical practice in gastroenterology and heptology.

Satish Keshav

Acknowledgements

I thank all the staff at Blackwell Publishing, particularly Geraldine Jeffers and Fiona Goodgame who were endlessly patient, enthusiastic and supportive. My students and colleagues provided inspiration, pertinent questions and useful comments. I also thank Michael Stein, who suggested this book, and Camilla and Vijay, who helped me to complete it.

List of abbreviations

ACh	acetylcholine
AFP	α-fetoprotein
AIDS	acquired immune deficiency syndrome
ALP	alkaline phosphatase
ALT	alanine transaminase
ANCA	antineutrophil cytoplasmic antibodies
5ASA	5-aminosalicylic acid
ASCA	antibodies to *Saccharomyces cerevisiae*
AST	aspartate transaminase
ATP	adenosine triphosphate
ATPase	adenosine triphosphatase
BAT	bile acid transporter
BEE	basal energy expenditure
BMI	body mass index
BMR	basal metabolic rate
BSE	bovine spongiform encephalopathy
Ca^{2+}	ionized calcium
cAMP	cyclic adenosine 3′,5′-cyclic monophosphate
CCK	cholecystokinin
CD	Crohn's disease
CEA	carcino-embryonic antigen
CFTR	cystic fibrosis transmembrane regulator
cGMP	cyclic guanosine monophosphate
CGRP	calcitonin gene-related peptide
Cl^-	chloride ion
CO_2	carbon dioxide
CoA	coenzyme A
CRC	colorectal cancer
CRP	C-reactive protein
CT	computerized tomography
CTZ	chemoreceptor trigger zone
DA	dopamine
DMT	divalent metal transporter
DNA	deoxyribonucleic acid
ECL	entero-chromaffin-like
EHEC	enterohaemorrhagic *Escherichia coli*
EPEC	enteropathogenic *Escherichia coli*
ERCP	endoscopic retrograde cholangiopancreatography
ESR	erythrocyte sedimentation rate
ETEC	enterotoxigenic *Escherichia coli*
FAP	familial adenomatous polyposis
Fe^{2+}	ferrous iron
Fe^{3+}	ferric iron
GABA	γ-amino butyric acid
γGT	γ-glutamyl transferase
H^+	ionized hydrogen
H_2O	water
H2R	histamine receptor type 2
HCG	human chorionic gonadotrophin
HCl	hydrochloric acid
HDL	high-density lipoproteins
5-HIAA	5-hydroxindole acetic acid
HIV	human immunodeficiency virus
HNPCC	hereditary non-polyposis colon cancer
5HT	5-hydroxytryptamine
IBD	inflammatory bowel disease
IBS	irritable bowel syndrome
IF	intrinsic factor
Ig	immunoglobulin
IL	interleukin
IMMC	interdigestive migrating motor complex
IPSID	immunoproliferative small intestinal disease
K^+	ionized potassium
LPS	lipopolysaccharide
MAD-CAM	mucosal addressin-cell adhesion molecule
MEN	multiple endocrine neoplasia
Mg^{2+}	ionized magnesium
MHC	major histocompatibility complex
MOAT	multispecific organic anion transporter
MRA	magnetic resonance angiography
MRCP	magnetic resonance cholangiopancreatography
MRI	magnetic resonance imaging
NA	noradrenaline
Na^+	ionized sodium
NAPQI	*N*-acetyl-*p*-benzoquinone-imine
NO	nitric oxide
NSAIDs	non-steroidal anti-inflammatory drugs
OAT	organic acid transport
PBC	primary biliary cirrhosis
PET	positron emission tomography
pIgA	polymeric immunoglobulin A
POMC	pro-opiomelanocortin
PSC	primary sclerosing cholangitis
PT	prothrombin time
PY	peptide Y
RNA	ribonucleic acid
SBP	spontaneous bacterial peritonitis
SC	secretory component
SGLT	sodium–glucose co-transporter
sIgA	secretory dimeric immunoglobulin A
STa	heat-stable enterotoxin
TECK	thymus and epithelial expressed chemokine
TGFβ	transforming growth factor β
TIPSS	transjugular intrahepatic portosystemic shunt
TNFα	tumour necrosis factor α
TPN	total parenteral nutrition
tTG	tissue transglutaminase
UC	ulcerative colitis
USS	ultrasound scanning
VC	vomiting centre
VIP	vasoactive intestinal peptide
VLDL	very low-density lipoproteins
WHO	World Health Organization

Introduction and overview

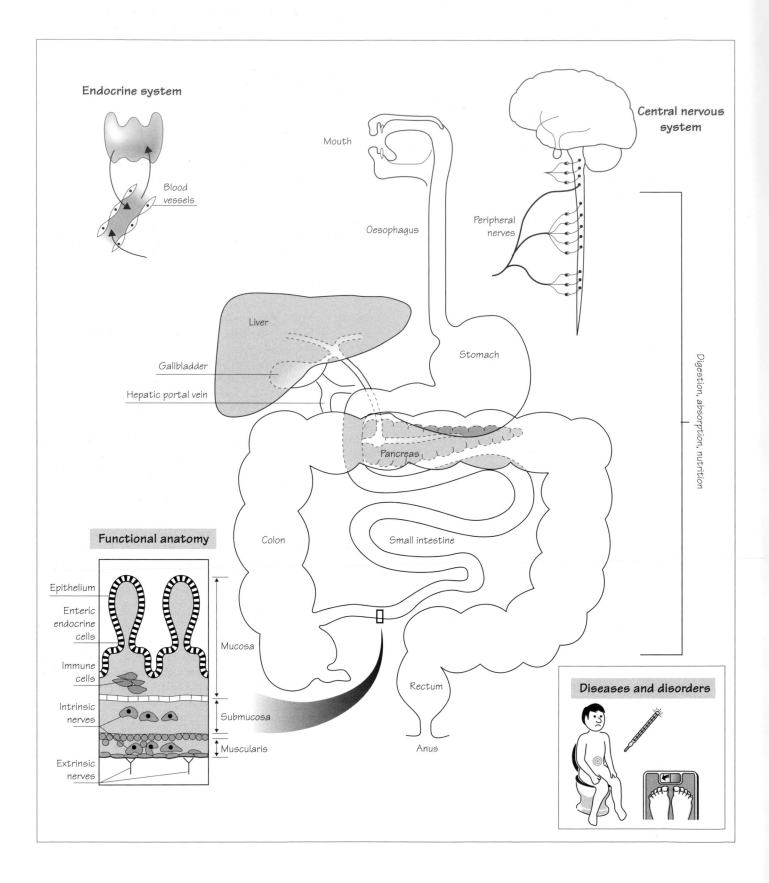

Endocrine system

Blood vessels

Mouth

Oesophagus

Central nervous system

Peripheral nerves

Liver

Gallbladder

Hepatic portal vein

Stomach

Pancreas

Colon

Small intestine

Digestion, absorption, nutrition

Functional anatomy

Epithelium

Enteric endocrine cells

Immune cells

Intrinsic nerves

Extrinsic nerves

Mucosa

Submucosa

Muscularis

Rectum

Anus

Diseases and disorders

Structure and function

The gastrointestinal system comprises the hollow organs from mouth to anus that form the gastrointestinal tract, the pancreas, which mainly secretes digestive juices into the small intestine, and the liver and biliary system, which perform vital metabolic functions in addition to their contribution to digestion and absorption of nutrients.

The intestinal tract

A hollow tubular structure into which nutrient-rich food is coerced, and from which wastes are expelled, is found in the most primitive multicellular organisms, from the hydra onwards. In humans, the tract is highly specialized throughout, both structurally and functionally. The mouth and teeth are the first structures in this tract and are connected by a powerful muscular tube, the oesophagus, to the stomach. The stomach stores food after meals and is the site where major digestive processes commence. The small intestine is the main digestive and absorptive surface. The large intestine acts mainly as a reservoir for food waste and allows reabsorption of water from the mainly liquid material leaving the small intestine. It is not essential for life and, paradoxically, is affected by a number of common, serious diseases, such as inflammatory bowel disease and colorectal cancer.

The pancreas

Digestive enzymes are produced in many parts of the gastrointestinal tract, including the mouth (salivary glands) and small intestine (enterocytes), although the exocrine pancreas is the most prodigious producer of digestive enzymes. Pancreatic failure causes malabsorption, which can be reversed by artificial enzyme supplements.

The liver and biliary system

Without the liver, survival is measured in hours, and no artificial system has yet been devised to substitute for hepatic function. The liver is the largest solid organ in the body and its essential functions include regulation of protein, fat and carbohydrate metabolism, synthesis of plasma proteins, ketones and lipoproteins, and detoxification and excretion. Via the hepatic portal circulation it receives and filters the entire venous drainage of the spleen, gastrointestinal tract and pancreas. Through the production of bile, it is also essential for digestion and absorption, particularly of dietary fats and fat-soluble vitamins.

Integrated function

The gastrointestinal system is controlled by both intrinsic and extrinsic neuronal and endocrine mechanisms. Enteric nerves and endocrine cells are particularly important in coordinating motility, digestion and absorption, and in regulating feeding and overall nutrition, including the control of body weight.

The gastrointestinal system presents a huge surface area that has to be protected against injury, particularly from microbial pathogens that are ingested with food and from the large population of commensal bacteria that populate the intestine. The mucosal immune system is critically important in regulating how the intestine responds to these challenges, providing protection and not reacting inappropriately to normal components of the diet.

Diseases and disorders

Nausea, vomiting, diarrhoea and constipation are common symptoms and their basic pathophysiology illustrates important aspects of gastrointestinal function.

Gastrointestinal symptoms are frequently not associated with any discernible pathological abnormality. These medically unexplained symptoms are often labelled functional disorders and, as our understanding of gastrointestinal physiology becomes more sophisticated, we may discover new explanations and treatments that are more effective.

Gastrointestinal system infections are common and are associated with significant morbidity and mortality worldwide. They range from self-limiting food poisoning to life-threatening local and systemic infections. Even peptic ulceration is most frequently caused by infection, with the *Helicobacter pylori* bacterium.

For some major diseases, such as inflammatory bowel disease, the aetiological agent has not been identified, despite rapidly advancing genetic and molecular research. Conversely, coeliac disease, another serious and common gastrointestinal inflammatory disease, is caused by a well-characterized immune response to wheat-derived proteins.

Colon cancer is a major cause of cancer-related death and our molecular and cellular understanding of its pathogenesis, and the pathophysiology of other gastrointestinal, pancreatic and liver tumours, is rapidly increasing.

Liver damage is often caused by infections or drugs and may be acute or chronic. Acute liver disease can rapidly progress to liver failure, or can resolve, either spontaneously or with appropriate treatment. Chronic liver disease may cause cirrhosis, which is characterized by a variety of signs and symptoms and changes throughout the body, including the effects of hepatic portal venous hypertension.

The gastrointestinal system is essential to nutrition, and disordered nutrition is a major issue worldwide – both through undernutrition and starvation and through overnutrition, which causes obesity, possibly the single most important modern health problem in the affluent world.

Diagnosis and treatment

Clinical assessment, including a focused history and examination, is the foundation of diagnosis. In addition, the gastrointestinal system can be investigated by endoscopy, radiology and specific functional tests. Endoscopy and radiology may also be used therapeutically, and pharmacotherapy and surgery for gastrointestinal disorders exploit many unique features of the structure and function of the system.

1 Mouth and teeth

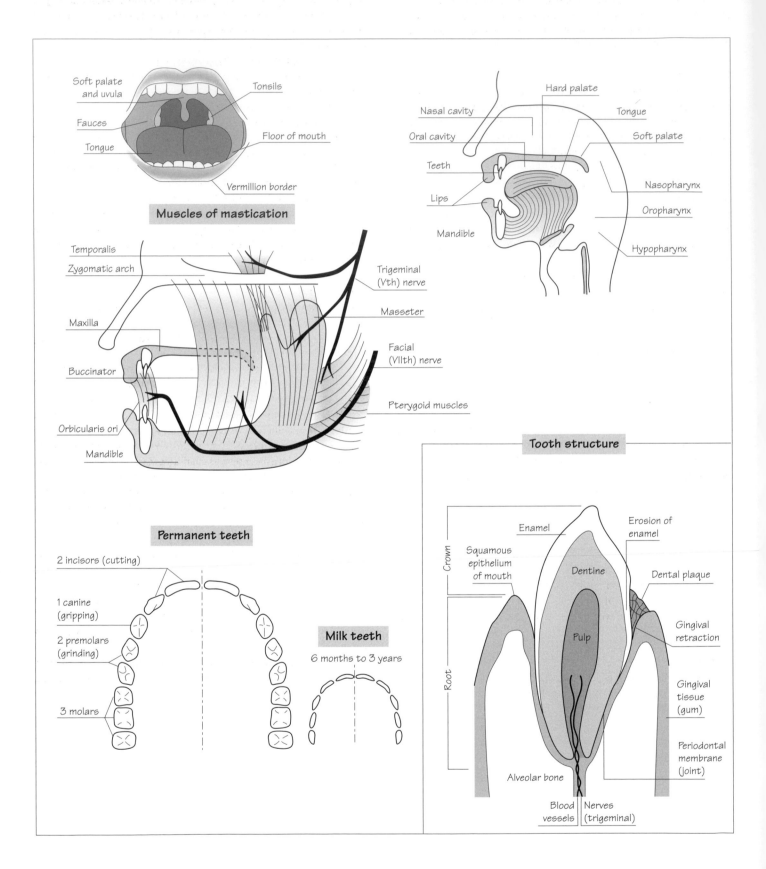

Soft palate and uvula

Tonsils

Fauces

Tongue

Floor of mouth

Vermillion border

Nasal cavity

Hard palate

Oral cavity

Tongue

Teeth

Soft palate

Lips

Nasopharynx

Mandible

Oropharynx

Hypopharynx

Muscles of mastication

Temporalis

Zygomatic arch

Trigeminal (Vth) nerve

Maxilla

Masseter

Buccinator

Facial (VIIth) nerve

Orbicularis ori

Pterygoid muscles

Mandible

Permanent teeth

2 incisors (cutting)

1 canine (gripping)

2 premolars (grinding)

3 molars

Milk teeth

6 months to 3 years

Tooth structure

Enamel

Erosion of enamel

Crown

Squamous epithelium of mouth

Dentine

Dental plaque

Pulp

Gingival retraction

Root

Gingival tissue (gum)

Alveolar bone

Periodontal membrane (joint)

Blood vessels

Nerves (trigeminal)

The mouth and teeth admit food into the gastrointestinal tract. They cut and break large pieces, chop, grind and moisten what can be chewed, and prepare a smooth, round bolus that can be swallowed and passed on to the rest of the system. Of course, the lips and mouth also serve other functions.

Structure

The sensitive, flexible, muscular **lips** that form the anterior border of the mouth can assess food by palpation, and their flexibility enables them to seal off the oral cavity and form variously a funnel, suction tube or shallow ladle to ingest fluids and food of varying consistency. The main muscles of the lips are **orbicularis ori**.

The **maxilla** and **mandible** support the roof and floor of the mouth, respectively. The arch of the mandible supports a sling of muscles that forms the floor, including the tongue. The maxilla is continuous with the rest of the skull and forms the roof of the mouth anteriorly and, simultaneously, the floor of the nasal cavity and paranasal **maxillary sinus**. Posteriorly, the roof is formed by the **soft palate**, composed of cartilage and connective tissue.

The sides of the mouth comprise the cheek muscles, chiefly **buccinator**, and supporting connective tissue. Posteriorly, the oral cavity opens into the oropharynx and the **tonsils** are situated between the **fauces** laterally, marking the posterior limit of the oral cavity.

The entire mouth, including the **gingivae** or gums, is lined with a tough, **non-cornified stratified squamous epithelium**, which changes to skin (cornified stratified squamous epithelium) at the **vermillion border** of the lips.

Teeth arise in the **alveolar bone** of the mandible and maxilla. Infants are born without external teeth and with precursors within the jaw. A transient set of 20 'milk' teeth erupts through the surface of the bone between 6 months and 2 years of age. They are shed between 6 and 13 years of age and permanent teeth take their place. There are 32 **permanent teeth** and the posterior molars, also known as wisdom teeth, may only erupt in young adulthood.

Teeth are living structures with a **vascular and nerve supply** (derived from the **trigeminal**, or IIIrd cranial, nerve) in the centre of each tooth, which is termed the **pulp**. Surrounding the pulp is a bony layer called **dentine** and surrounding this is an extremely hard, calcified layer called **enamel**. Teeth lie in sockets within the alveolar bone and the joint is filled with a layer of tough fibrous tissue (the **periodontal membrane**) allowing a small amount of flexibility. The margins of the tooth joint are surrounded by **gingivae**, which are a continuation of the mucosal lining of the mouth.

Function

The lips, cheeks and tongue help to keep food moving and place it in the optimal position for effective chewing. The main muscles of chewing or mastication are the **masseter** and **temporalis**, which powerfully bring the lower jaw up against the upper jaw, and the **pterygoids**, which open the jaws, keep them aligned, and moves them sideways, and backwards, and forwards for grinding. The trigeminal (Vth cranial) nerve controls the muscles of mastication.

Teeth are specialized for different tasks as follows:
- **Incisors** have flat, sharp edges for cutting tough foods, such as meat and hard fruits.
- **Canines** have pointed, sharp ends for gripping food, particularly meat, and tearing away pieces.
- **Premolars** and **molars** have flattened, complex surfaces that capture tiny bits of food, such as grains, and allow them to be crushed between the surfaces of two opposed teeth. As people get older, the grinding surfaces of the molars are gradually worn down.

Certain **drugs** can be absorbed across the oral mucosa and may be prescribed **sublingually** (under the tongue). In this way, the need to swallow is avoided and the absorbed drug bypasses the liver and avoids hepatic first-pass metabolism. **Glyceryl trinitrate** is one of the most common drugs administered in this way.

Common disorders

Herpes simplex infection of the mouth is very common, causing **cold sores**, which often erupt on the lips when people have other illnesses. Serious oral infections, usually caused by a mixture of anaerobic bacteria, are less common.

The corners of the mouth may be ulcerated or fissured in patients who cannot take care of their mouths, for example after a stroke, so careful oral hygiene is important in these cases. Nutritional deficiency, particularly of B complex vitamins and iron, is also associated with fissures at the edge of the mouth, known as **angular stomatitis**.

Shallow 'apthous' ulcers in the mouth are common and are usually not associated with a more serious condition. Rarely squamous cell carcinoma can develop. Risk factors include smoking and chewing tobacco or betel nut, which is particularly common on the Indian subcontinent.

Dental caries is the commonest disorder of teeth, resulting in tooth loss with advancing age. It is caused by chronic bacterial infection of the gums and periodontal membrane, encouraged by carbohydrate and **sugar-rich food residues** left in the mouth. **Bacteria** grow in the gap between the tooth enamel and gums, forming a hard, impenetrable layer called **plaque**, within which they multiply. Their metabolic products, including **organic acids**, damage tooth enamel. Gradual erosion of enamel and retraction of the gingivae weakens the tooth joint. Infection can penetrate the pulp causing an **abscess**, and chronic infection can destroy and devitalize the pulp.

Dental hygiene, including brushing and flossing and having **fluoride** in drinking water, which strengthens tooth enamel, reduces the incidence of caries.

2 Salivary glands

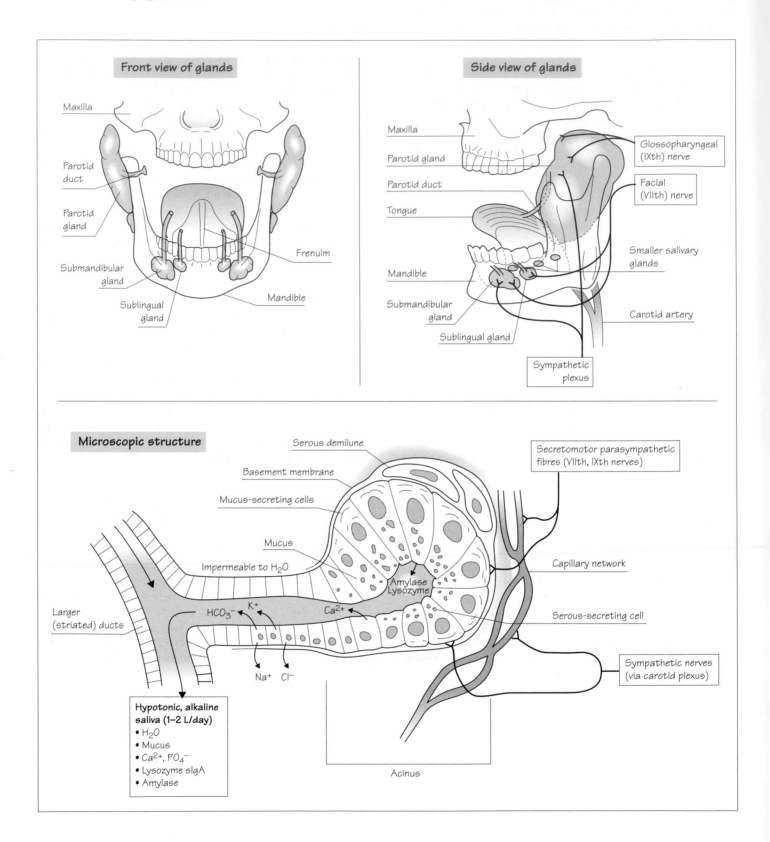

Front view of glands

- Maxilla
- Parotid duct
- Parotid gland
- Submandibular gland
- Sublingual gland
- Frenulm
- Mandible

Side view of glands

- Maxilla
- Parotid gland
- Parotid duct
- Tongue
- Mandible
- Submandibular gland
- Sublingual gland
- Glossopharyngeal (IXth) nerve
- Facial (VIIth) nerve
- Smaller salivary glands
- Carotid artery
- Sympathetic plexus

Microscopic structure

- Serous demilune
- Basement membrane
- Mucus-secreting cells
- Mucus
- Impermeable to H$_2$O
- Amylase Lysozyme
- Larger (striated) ducts
- HCO$_3$$^-$
- K$^+$
- Ca^{2+}
- Na$^+$ Cl$^-$
- Secretomotor parasympathetic fibres (VIIth, IXth nerves)
- Capillary network
- Serous-secreting cell
- Sympathetic nerves (via carotid plexus)
- Acinus

Hypotonic, alkaline saliva (1–2 L/day)
- H$_2$O
- Mucus
- Ca^{2+}, PO$_4$$^-$
- Lysozyme sIgA
- Amylase

Saliva lubricates the mouth and teeth, provides antibacterial and digestive enzymes, and maintains the chemical balance of tooth enamel. Salivary glands are structurally similar to exocrine glands throughout the gastrointestinal tract and are also regulated in a typical way.

Structure

The three main pairs of salivary glands are the **parotid**, **submandibular** and **sublingual** glands and there are many smaller, unnamed glands lining the mouth. The larger glands have main ducts that transport the saliva to the oral cavity.

The parotid gland is the largest, situated on the side of the face, in front of the ears and below the zygomatic arch. The facial nerve courses through the parotid gland. The parotid duct enters the mouth opposite the second molar teeth.

The submandibular gland is situated medial to the body of the mandible and the sublingual glands lie medial to the submandibular glands. The duct of the submandibular gland opens onto the mouth at the side of the base of the tongue.

Microscopically, salivary glands typify the structure of **exocrine** glands throughout the body. They are **lobulated**, with fibrous **septae** or partitions between **lobules**. The functional unit is the spherical **acinus**, which comprises a single layer of secretory epithelial cells around the central lumen.

The secretory cells are **pyramidal** shaped, with the base resting on the basement membrane and the tip towards the lumen. The cell's synthetic machinery, comprising of endoplasmic reticulum and ribosomes, is located near the base and the protein-exporting machinery, comprising of golgi apparatus and **secretory vesicles**, is located in the apical portion. Nuclei are located centrally. Serous cells tend to have small dense apical granules, while mucus-secreting cells tend to be more columnar and have larger, pale-staining apical granules.

The secretory epithelium merges with the epithelial lining of **ductules**, which coalesce to form progressively larger **ducts** that convey saliva to the surface.

Most secretory cells in salivary gland acini are **seromucoid**, secreting a thick mucoid fluid that also contains proteins. Some cells secrete a watery, serous fluid, while others secrete predominantly mucoid material. Acini with mainly mucus-secreting cells also have **serous demilunes** lying just outside the main acinus and within the basement membrane. The parotid gland secretes the most watery saliva and most acini in this gland are composed entirely of serous cells, while the submandibular and sublingual glands secrete a more viscid mucus saliva.

The **facial** (VIIth cranial) and **glossopharyngeal** (IXth cranial) nerves supply secretomotor parasympathetic fibres from the **salivary nuclei** in the brainstem, and **sympathetic** nerves are derived from the cervical sympathetic chain.

Function

One to two litres of saliva are secreted each day and almost all is swallowed and reabsorbed. Secretion is under **autonomic** control. Food in the mouth stimulates nerve fibres that end in the **nucleus of the tractus solitarius** and, in turn, stimulate salivary nuclei in the mid-brain. Salivation is also stimulated by sight, smell and anticipation of food through impulses from the cortex acting on **brainstem salivary nuclei**. Intense sympathetic activity inhibits saliva production, which is why nervous anxiety causes a dry mouth. Similarly, drugs that inhibit parasympathetic nerve activity, such as some antidepressants, tranquillizers and opiate analgesics, can cause dry mouth (**xerostomia**).

Saliva, composed of water and mucins, forms a gel-like coating over the oral mucosa and **lubricates** food. Lubrication is essential for **chewing** and the formation of a bolus of food that can be easily **swallowed**. Saliva also dissolves chemicals in food and allows them to interact more efficiently with taste buds. **Taste** is an important sense as it allows us to choose nutritious foods and to avoid unpleasant tasting foods that may be harmful, or to which we have developed an aversion as a result of previous experience.

Saliva also contains α-amylase, which begins the process of carbohydrate digestion, although its overall contribution is probably minor.

Saliva contains **antibacterial enzymes**, such as lysozyme, and **immunoglobulins** that may help to prevent serious infection, and maintain control of the resident bacterial flora of the mouth.

Salivary duct cells are relatively impermeable to water and secrete K^+, HCO_3^-, Ca^{2+}, Mg^{2+}, phosphate ions and water, so that the final product of salivary gland secretion is a hypotonic, **alkaline** fluid that is rich in **calcium and phosphate**. This composition is important to prevent **demineralization** of tooth **enamel**.

Common disorders

Anticholinergic drugs are the most common cause of decreased saliva production and dry mouth, also known as **xerostomia**. Less common causes include autoimmune damage to salivary glands in **Sjogren's** syndrome and sarcoidosis. Xerostomia is a serious condition, because chewing and swallowing rely on adequate saliva, as does maintaining teeth in good condition.

Occasionally **stones** can form in the salivary glands, causing obstruction, pain and swelling in the proximal part of the gland.

The **mumps** virus, for unknown reasons, preferentially attacks the salivary glands, pancreas, ovaries and testicles, and parotid inflammation causes the typical swollen cheeks appearance of mumps.

3 Tongue and pharynx

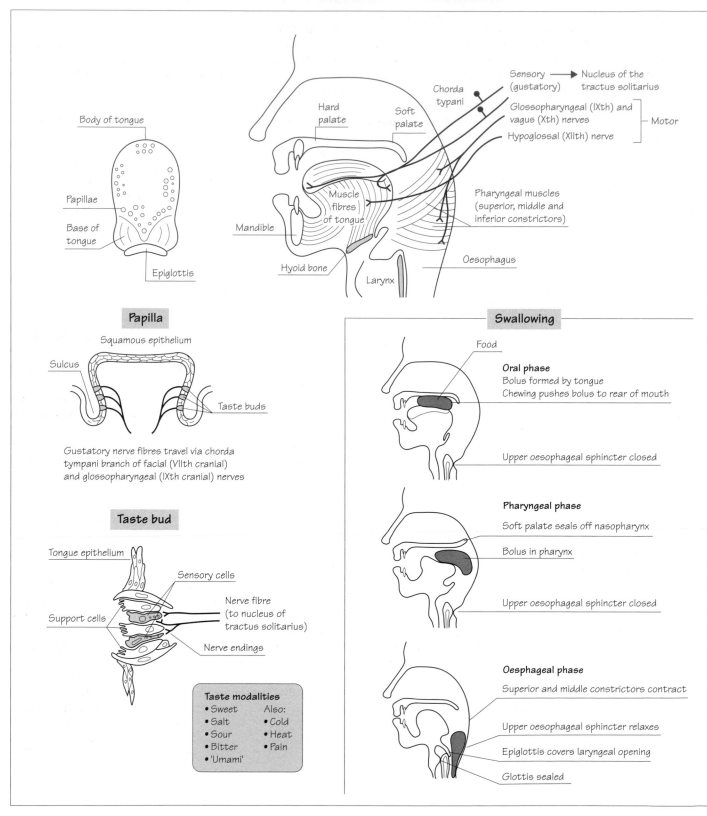

Body of tongue

Papillae

Base of tongue

Epiglottis

Hard palate

Soft palate

Chorda typani

Sensory (gustatory) → Nucleus of the tractus solitarius

Glossopharyngeal (IXth) and vagus (Xth) nerves

Hypoglossal (XIIth) nerve

Motor

Muscle fibres of tongue

Pharyngeal muscles (superior, middle and inferior constrictors)

Mandible

Oesophagus

Hyoid bone

Larynx

Papilla

Squamous epithelium

Sulcus

Taste buds

Gustatory nerve fibres travel via chorda tympani branch of facial (VIIth cranial) and glossopharyngeal (IXth cranial) nerves

Taste bud

Tongue epithelium

Sensory cells

Nerve fibre (to nucleus of tractus solitarius)

Support cells

Nerve endings

Taste modalities
- Sweet   Also:
- Salt   • Cold
- Sour   • Heat
- Bitter   • Pain
- 'Umami'

Swallowing

Food

Oral phase
Bolus formed by tongue
Chewing pushes bolus to rear of mouth

Upper oesophageal sphincter closed

Pharyngeal phase

Soft palate seals off nasopharynx

Bolus in pharynx

Upper oesophageal sphincter closed

Oesophageal phase

Superior and middle constrictors contract

Upper oesophageal sphincter relaxes

Epiglottis covers laryngeal opening

Glottis sealed

The tongue and taste buds are an essential part of the mouth, involved in taste, chewing, talking and many other functions.

The tongue

The tongue is a powerful, mobile, muscular organ attached to the mandible and hyoid bone. The body is a flat, oblong surface with a longitudinal ridge along the top. It lies on the floor of the mouth and a thin membranous **frenulum** runs along the under surface in the mid-line anteriorly. Posteriorly, the root is formed from muscle fibres passing downward towards the pharynx and the epiglottis forms its posterior border.

The tongue is covered with a tough non-cornified stratified **squamous epithelium** continuous with the rest of the oral mucosa. On its upper surface it is thrown up into numerous **ridges and papillae**, creating a roughened surface to rasp and lick food. Papillae around the lateral and posterior edges contain numerous **taste buds**. These contain specialized **sensory cells** that communicate directly with **nerve endings** from sensory nerve dendrites. The sensory cells are surrounded and supported by adjacent epithelial cells. They express receptors for chemicals dissolved in **saliva** and each taste bud is sensitive to a single major modality.

The **hypoglossal** (XIIth cranial) **nerve** innervates the tongue muscle. Sensory fibres travel in the **glossopharyngeal** (IXth cranial) nerve and in the **chorda tympani** branch of the **facial** (VIIth cranial) nerve. Taste fibres terminate in the **nucleus of the tractus solitarius** in the mid-brain. The tongue also has a large representation in the **somatic** motor and sensory **cortex** of the brain.

Function

The tongue moves in all planes and reaches throughout the mouth. It **directs** food between the teeth, **retrieves** pieces stuck between the teeth and **clears** away obstructions. It **propels** food and drink posteriorly to initiate the pharyngeal phase of swallowing. The tongue is also crucial to **speech**, varying its shape and selectively closing off and opening air channels.

The major modalities of taste are **sweet**, **sour**, **salt** and **bitter**, and a fifth modality, called **umami**, typified by monosodium glutamate, is now also recognized. Taste **receptors** include G-protein-coupled receptors, ion channels and **cold**, **heat** and **pain** receptors. The flavour of food is a combination of taste and **smell**, which is sensed by a large family of G-protein-coupled olfactory receptors that bind to a myriad of different chemicals.

Common disorders

The tongue may be **paralyzed** by damage to the hypoglossal nerve or a stroke affecting its central connections. In **motor neuron disease**, spontaneous **fasciculations** are readily seen in the denervated tongue muscle.

The tongue may be affected by squamous cell carcinoma and herpes simplex infection (see Chapter 1). Occasionally the tongue may be pigmented, which is not pathological. **Glossitis**, manifest by a smooth, red, swollen, painful tongue occurs; for example, with B-vitamin deficiencies.

Dry mouth, or **xerostomia**, affects taste profoundly, as chemicals must be dissolved for the taste buds to function. Systemic diseases, such as **uraemia**, and drugs, such as **metronidazole**, may **alter taste** by interfering with the function of taste buds.

The pharynx

The pharynx is an air-filled cavity at the back of the nose and mouth, above the openings of the larynx and oesophagus. The walls of the oropharynx are lined by the same non-cornified stratified **squamous epithelium** that lines the oral cavity.

Superiorly, the floor of the sphenoidal air sinus and the skull base bound the **nasopharynx**. The soft palate can be drawn up, closing the connection between the nasopharynx and oropharynx.

The **oropharynx** is bounded posteriorly by tissues overlying the bodies of the upper cervical vertebrae and laterally by the **tonsils** and the openings of the **Eustachian tubes**, which connect the pharynx with the middle ear. Inferiorly it narrows into the **hypopharynx**.

Three straps of voluntary muscle surround the pharynx, overlapping each other and forming the **superior, middle and inferior constrictors**. The circular muscle of the upper oesophagus is continuous with the inferior constrictor.

Motor and sensory fibres mainly travel in the **glossopharyngeal** (IXth cranial) and **vagus** (Xth cranial) nerves.

Function

The pharynx is a conduit for air, food and drink, and **swallowing** requires coordinated action of the tongue, pharyngeal, laryngeal and oesophageal muscles, and is controlled by the **brainstem**, via the glossopharyngeal and trigeminal nerves.

The tongue forces a bolus of food backwards into the **oropharynx**, initiating a reflex that raises the soft palate, sealing off the **nasopharynx**, and inhibits respiration.

The superior and middle pharyngeal constrictors force the bolus down into the **hypopharynx**, and the **glottis** closes. The **epiglottis** is forced backwards and downwards, forming a chute over the **larynx**, opening onto the upper oesophageal sphincter.

The sphincter relaxes, allowing the bolus to enter the oesophagus. It is then conveyed downwards by peristalsis. The glottis reopens and respiration recommences.

Common disorders

The pharynx is critically important in ensuring that the upper airway is protected from **aspiration** of food, saliva and drink during swallowing and vomiting. Thus neurological disorders, including **stroke**, **motor neuron disease**, **myasthenia gravis** or reduced conscious level associated with **intoxication**, **anaesthesia** or **coma** can cause **aspiration** into the lungs, and **pneumonia**.

Upper respiratory tract infections often cause **pharyngitis** and may cause **tonsillitis**. Common pathogens include viruses, such as **influenza** and the Epstein–Barr virus, and bacteria, such as **streptococci**. Group A β-haemolytic streptococci may also cause **rheumatic fever**, a systemic autoimmune disorder that can affect the skin, heart and brain. **Diphtheria** is a serious cause of pharyngitis that is preventable by immunization.

4 Oesophagus

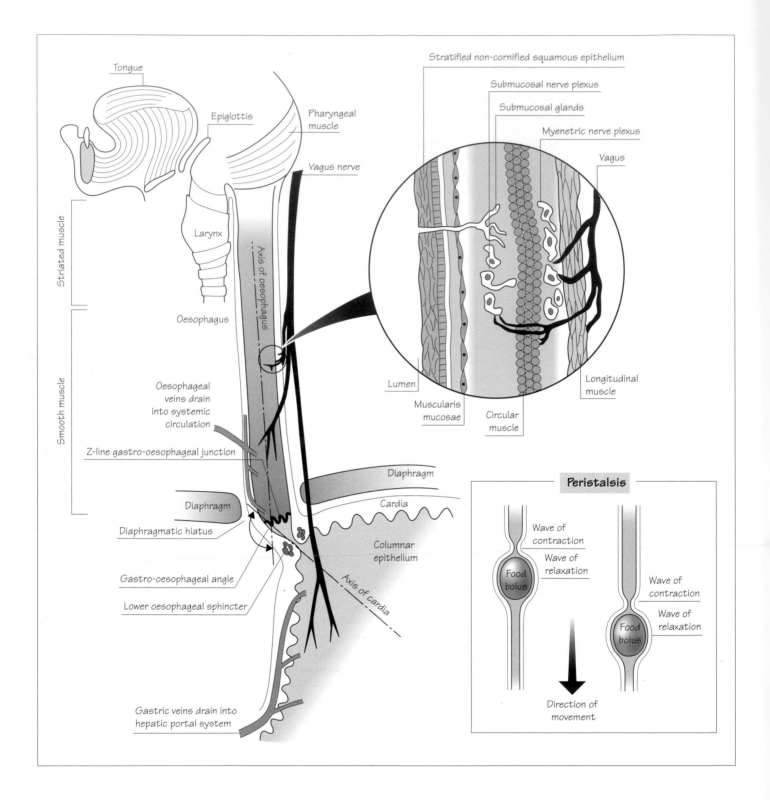

Tongue

Epiglottis

Pharyngeal muscle

Vagus nerve

Larynx

Oesophagus

Axis of oesophagus

Striated muscle

Smooth muscle

Oesophageal veins drain into systemic circulation

Z-line gastro-oesophageal junction

Diaphragm

Diaphragm

Diaphragmatic hiatus

Gastro-oesophageal angle

Lower oesophageal sphincter

Gastric veins drain into hepatic portal system

Cardia

Columnar epithelium

Axis of cardia

Stratified non-cornified squamous epithelium

Submucosal nerve plexus

Submucosal glands

Myenetric nerve plexus

Vagus

Lumen

Muscularis mucosae

Circular muscle

Longitudinal muscle

Peristalsis

Wave of contraction

Wave of relaxation

Food bolus

Wave of contraction

Wave of relaxation

Food bolus

Direction of movement

The oesophagus carries food and liquid from the mouth to the stomach and the rest of the intestinal tract and is an important site of common gastrointestinal disorders.

Structure

The oesophagus is a muscular tube, beginning at the **pharynx** and ending at the **stomach**. It traverses the neck and **thorax**, where it lies close to the trachea, the great vessels and the left atrium of the heart. The upper opening of the oesophagus lies behind the opening of the larynx and is separated from it by the arytenoid folds. The **epiglottis**, attached to the back of the tongue, can flap over the larynx, protecting it during swallowing and funnelling food towards the oesophagus. Just above the gastro-oesophageal junction, the oesophagus traverses a natural **hiatus** or gap in the **diaphragm**, to enter the abdomen.

The walls of the oesophagus reflect the general organization of the intestinal wall. The walls are formed from outside to inside by:
- adventitia or serosa;
- longitudinal muscle layer;
- circular muscle layer;
- submucosal layer;
- muscularis mucosae;
- mucosa and epithelium.

The muscle in the upper third is **striated** muscle and in the lower two-thirds, **smooth** muscle similar to the rest of the gut. The lower oesophageal muscle remains in tonic contraction and forms part of the **lower oesophageal sphincter**. The **angulation** of the oesophagus as it enters the stomach and the diaphragmatic muscle help to keep the lower oesophagus closed.

The **vagus** nerve runs alongside the oesophagus and innervates oesophageal muscle directly and via intrinsic nerves in the **myenteric nerve plexus** located between the longitudinal and circular muscle layers, and the **submucosal plexus**.

The submucosa contains lobulated **glands** that secrete lubricating material through small ducts that penetrate the epithelial surface.

The oesophageal epithelium is a tough, non-cornified **stratified squamous** epithelium, which changes abruptly to a non-stratified columnar epithelium at the **gastro-oesophageal junction**, known as the **Z-line**.

Importantly, venous drainage of the oesophagus forms a **submucosal venous plexus** that drains directly into the systemic venous circulation, avoiding the hepatic portal vein and liver. This plexus anastomoses with veins in the stomach that drain into the **hepatic portal system**. In portal hypertension, collateral veins divert gastric blood to the oesophageal veins, which enlarge and form **varices**.

Function

The oesophagus conveys food, drink and saliva from the pharynx to the stomach, by **peristalsis**. Peristalsis comprises a coordinated wave of contraction behind the bolus of food, with relaxation ahead of it, propelling the food bolus forward. It is involuntary, resulting from intrinsic neuromuscular reflexes in the intestinal wall, independent of extrinsic innervation. However, external stimuli modify the frequency and strength of peristaltic activity throughout the intestine. Very strong peristaltic contractions can cause pain.

In **vomiting**, peristaltic waves travel in the reverse direction, propelling food upward towards the mouth.

Common disorders

Dysphagia is difficulty in swallowing and **odynophagia** is painful swallowing. Sensations arising from the oesophagus are usually felt **retrosternally** in the lower part of the centre of the chest. **Heartburn** describes a burning, unpleasant retrosternal sensation that may be caused by acid reflux from the stomach into the oesophagus.

Obstruction to flow down the oesophagus causes dysphagia and may be complete, halting swallowing altogether, so that the patient cannot even swallow saliva and **drools** continually. Chronic obstruction may lead to **aspiration** of food into the larynx, causing **pneumonia**. Refluxed stomach acid reaching the larynx can cause inflammation, causing cough and a hoarse voice.

Cancer of the oesophagus or trauma, caused, for example, by a fishbone, can create a **fistula** from the oesophagus to the trachea, which lies immediately anteriorly. This can lead to recurrent infection caused by bacteria in the oesophageal fluid (**aspiration pneumonia**).

The lower oesophageal sphincter is relatively weak; therefore, **acid reflux** is common even in health, but can be excessive, when it may cause **oesophagitis**. Chronic acid reflux can induce the epithelium to change from the normal squamous lining to a gastric or intestine-like columnar lining. This epithelial **metaplasia** is called **Barrett's** oesophagus and it increases the risk of developing adenocarcinoma of the oesophagus.

The diaphragmatic hiatus through which the oesophagus passes from the thorax to the abdomen widens with age and it may allow the upper part of the stomach to herniate into the thorax. This is known as a sliding **hiatus hernia**, which increases the risk of reflux oesophagitis. The sliding is aggravated by obesity and lying flat in bed (see Chapter 30).

Very powerful muscular contraction and peristalsis (**dysmotility**) can cause discomfort or pain. Progressive failure of peristalsis and a chronically hypertonic lower oesophageal sphincter, leading to a dilated, non-functioning oesophagus, is called **achalasia**.

Forceful retching or vomiting can cause a **Mallory–Weiss** tear in the oesophageal mucosa, which may bleed, causing (usually) self-limiting **haematemesis**. By contrast, oesophageal **varices** formed in portal hypertension can bleed catastrophically (see Chapter 10).

Infections of the oesophagus are rare. The most common is **candidiasis**, occurring in immunocompromised patients and those with diabetes mellitus.

Squamous carcinoma of the oesophagus is particularly common in southern Africa and may relate to diet, smoking and carcinogens in the soil, as well to genetic factors. **Adenocarcinoma**, arising from Barrett's oesophagus, is becoming more common in the Western world (see Chapter 38).

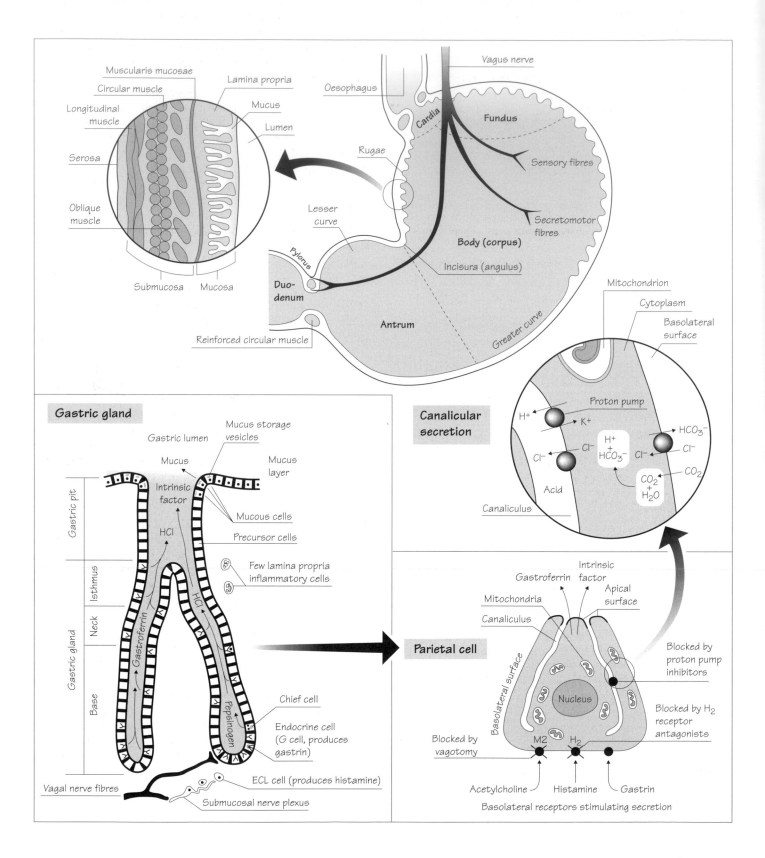

The stomach is the first wholly intra-abdominal intestinal organ. It is adapted for mechanical churning, storage and digestion of food and contributes to neuro-endocrine coordination of intestinal function. The basic rhythm of the intestine, the gastric slow wave, originates here.

Structure

The stomach is 'J'-shaped, with lesser and greater **curvatures**, facing to the right. The **spleen** lies to the left and the **pancreas** lies inferiorly and posteriorly. The **liver** lies to the right. The stomach lies behind the left hypochondrial region on the surface of the abdomen.

The stomach comprises five distinct regions:

1 the **cardia** immediately adjoining the oesophagus;
2 the dome-shaped **fundus** extending to the left of the **cardia**;
3 the body or **corpus**;
4 the **antrum**;
5 the **pylorus**, in which the circular muscle layer is reinforced, and which forms a tight sphincter separating the stomach from the duodenum.

The structure of the gastric wall reflects the general organization of hollow intestinal organs, with an additional **oblique muscle layer** that supports its mechanical churning function and allows it to expand. From outside to inside the walls are formed from:

• serosa;
• longitudinal muscle layer;
• circular muscle layer;
• oblique muscle layer;
• submucosa;
• muscularis mucosae;
• mucosa comprising the lamina propria and columnar gastric epithelium with its pits and glands.

The **coeliac** artery supplies arterial blood to the stomach and venous blood drains into the **hepatic portal vein**. The stomach receives parasympathetic nerves via the **vagus** (Xth cranial) nerve and sympathetic fibres from the splanchnic nerves.

Most of the gastric mucosa is thrown up in coarse folds called **rugae**, while the antral mucosa is much smoother. A thick **mucus** layer protects against mechanical trauma, HCl and proteolytic enzymes.

Gastric pits are narrow invaginations of the epithelium into the lamina propria. Two or three **gastric glands** are connected to each pit via a narrow **isthmus**, leading to the **neck** region of each gland. Gastric glands are tubular structures with specialized cells for the production of HCl (**parietal or oxyntic cells**) and pepsin (**chief cells**), as well as **mucus**-producing **goblet cells**, undifferentiated epithelial cells, **entero-endocrine** cells and stem cells.

Parietal cells are found in glands throughout the fundus, corpus and antrum. They secrete **HCl**, the glycoproteins **intrinsic factor** and **gastroferrin**, which facilitate the absorption of vitamin B_{12} and iron, respectively.

Chief cells are found predominantly in the corpus. They secrete **pepsinogen** and have an extensive rough endoplasmic reticulum and prominent apical secretory granules.

The main entero-endocrine cells of the stomach are **G cells**, producing **gastrin, D cells,** producing **somatostatin**, and **entero-chromaffin-like (ECL)** cells, producing **histamine** (see Chapter 16).

Function

Food is **mixed** thoroughly by the churning action of gastric muscle against a closed pyloric sphincter. The pylorus opens only to allow semi-liquid material (**chyme**) through into the duodenum, preventing the passage of large food particles. Mechanical dysruption increases the surface area for more efficient digestion and prevents damage to the delicate intestinal mucosa from large, hard, irregular food particles.

Rhythmic electric activity in the stomach produces regular peristaltic waves three times a minute, known as the **gastric slow wave**.

Gastric **secretion** is stimulated by the anticipation of food, the so-called **cephalic phase**, and by food reaching the stomach, the **gastric phase**. **Acetylcholine** and **histamine**, acting through **M2 muscarinic** and **H2 receptors** stimulate the secretion of HCl.

Parietal cells have an extensive intracellular **canalicular** system, numerous **mitochondria** to generate energy, and a highly active K^+/H^+ adenosine triphosphatase (ATPase) pump (**proton pump**) that secretes H^+ into the lumen. An apical chloride channel transports Cl^- into the lumen, to form **HCl**.

At the basolateral surface, HCO_3^-, formed intracellularly from CO_2 and H_2O, is exchanged for Cl^-, so that circulating HCO_3^- levels rise when the stomach secretes acid ('**alkali tide**'). The basolateral **Na+/K+ ATPase pump** also replenishes intracellular K^+ levels.

Differentiation and secretion of parietal cells is also stimulated by **gastrin**. Acid secretion is increased by excess gastrin, for example, in the **Zollinger–Ellison** syndrome (see Chapter 16), and is inhibited by **vagotomy**, which removes cholinergic stimulation, by H2 receptor antagonists, such as **ranitidine**, and by proton pump inhibitors, such as **omeprazole**, which irreversibly bind to the K^+/H^+ ATPase.

HCl activates **pepsinogen**, to produce pepsin, initiating protein digestion. **Intrinsic factor** binds to vitamin B_{12}, allowing it to escape degradation in the stomach and intestine and to be safely transported to the terminal ileum, where it is absorbed. Gastroferrin binds to Fe^{2+}, facilitating absorption in the duodenum (see Chapter 21).

Common disorders

Symptoms relating to the stomach are extremely common, but are frequently not caused by discernable organic disease (see Chapter 29). Typical symptoms include **nausea, epigastric pain** and **bloating**. Collectively these symptoms are termed **dyspepsia** and patients may refer to them as **indigestion**. With serious conditions of the stomach, there may also be **vomiting, haematemesis, melaena** and **loss of weight**.

The main serious gastric conditions are peptic **ulcer** and **gastritis**, which are most frequently associated with *Helicobacter pylori* infection and the use of non-steroidal anti-inflammatory drugs (**NSAIDs**), and gastric **carcinoma** (see Chapter 31).

Hiatus hernia occurs when part of the stomach herniates through the diaphragmatic hiatus through which the oesophagus passes (see Chapters 30 & 38). Gastric outlet **obstruction** may occur in young male infants, due to a congenitally hypertrophied sphincter, causing projectile vomiting. In adults, a more common cause is autonomic **neuropathy**, caused, for example, by **diabetes mellitus**.

6 Duodenum

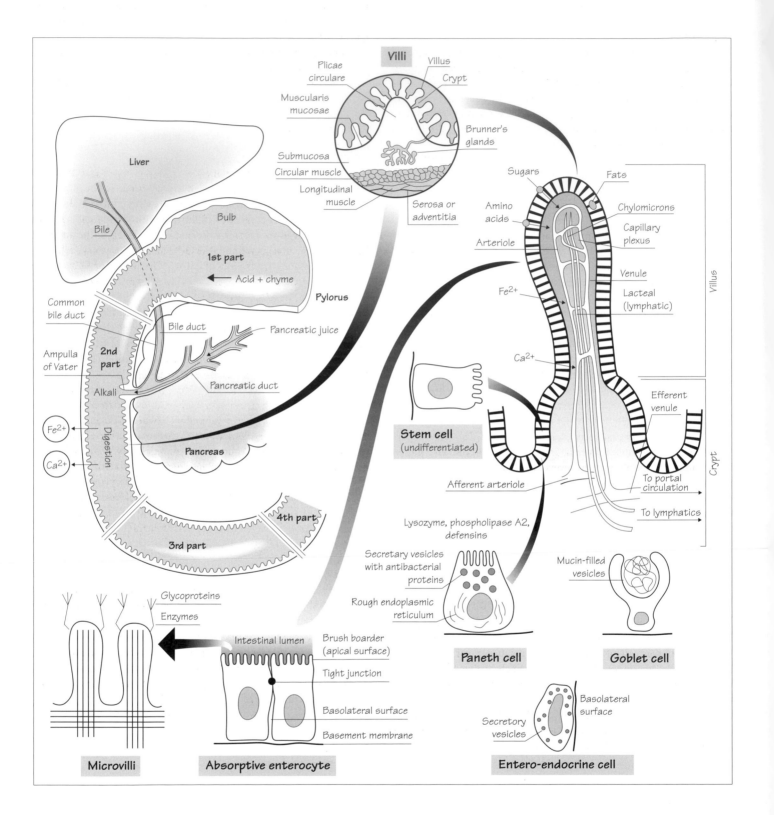

Villi

Plicae circulare
Villus
Crypt
Muscularis mucosae
Brunner's glands
Submucosa
Circular muscle
Longitudinal muscle
Serosa or adventitia

Liver
Bile
Bulb
1st part
← Acid + chyme
Pylorus
Common bile duct
Bile duct
Pancreatic juice
Ampulla of Vater
2nd part
Alkali
Pancreatic duct
Fe^{2+}
Digestion
Ca^{2+}
Pancreas
4th part
3rd part

Sugars
Fats
Amino acids
Chylomicrons
Arteriole
Capillary plexus
Fe^{2+}
Venule
Lacteal (lymphatic)
Ca^{2+}
Villus

Stem cell (undifferentiated)

Efferent venule
Afferent arteriole
To portal circulation
To lymphatics
Crypt

Lysozyme, phospholipase A2, defensins
Secretary vesicles with antibacterial proteins
Rough endoplasmic reticulum

Mucin-filled vesicles

Paneth cell
Goblet cell

Glycoproteins
Enzymes
Intestinal lumen
Brush boarder (apical surface)
Tight junction
Basolateral surface
Basement membrane

Basolateral surface
Secretory vesicles

Microvilli
Absorptive enterocyte
Entero-endocrine cell

The duodenum is the first major digestive and absorptive region of the intestine, receiving chyme from the stomach and mixing it with bile, pancreatic juice and enteric secretions.

Structure

The duodenum extends from the **pylorus**, to the jejunum at the **ligament of Treitz**. It is approximately 30 cm long and 'C'-shaped, facing the left, and is mostly **retroperitoneal**. The first part of the duodenum is called the **bulb**. The second part receives bile and pancreatic juice via the **ampulla of Vater** and lies adjacent to the **pancreas** on the left. The **coeliac** artery supplies the duodenum and venous drainage is via the **superior mesenteric vein** into the hepatic portal vein.

The walls of the duodenum reflect the general organization of the intestinal wall. They comprise from the outside to the inside:

- adventitia or serosa;
- longitudinal muscle layer;
- circular muscle layer;
- submucosa containing Brunner's glands;
- muscularis mucosae;
- mucosal layer comprising the lamina propria and epithelial lining.

The **epithelium** rests on a basement membrane, on the loose connective tissue of the **lamina propria**, which is thrown up into finger-like **villi** and is indented into long, thin **crypts** (of **Lieberkühn**) from which new epithelial cells emerge. A thin layer of smooth muscle, the **muscularis mucosa**, separates the mucosa from the **submucosa**, which is thrown up in transverse folds known as **plicae circulare**. Branched tubular glands, called **Brunner's glands**, are located in the submucosa and are connected to the lumen by narrow ducts. The lamina propria contains numerous fibroblasts, macrophages, lymphocytes, neutrophils, mast cells, vascular endothelial cells and other cells.

An **arteriole**, **venule** and a lymphatic channel called a **lacteal** supply each villus. The arteriole and venule form a **countercurrent circulation** enhancing intestinal absorption. Intrinsic **enteric nerves** ramify through the layers of the intestine, controlling motor and secretory function (see Chapter 17).

The small intestinal epithelium contains a number of distinct cell types, all of which differentiate from stem cells located in the crypt.

Enterocytes constitute most of the intestinal lining. They are columnar, with a round or oblong nucleus located centrally. On the luminal surface, **microvilli**, supported by an extensive network of cytoskeletal proteins, increase the surface area available for digestion and absorption. The surface of the microvilli are covered by glycoproteins and attached enzymes and mucins, forming a prominent **brush border**. **Tight junctions** link adjacent enterocytes, so that the apical surface of the cell, and consequently the luminal surface of the intestine, is isolated from the basal surface. Thus, gradients of nutrients and electrolytes can be maintained and pathogens can be excluded. Enterocytes synthesize digestive enzymes and secrete them to the apical brush border.

Goblet cells are specialized secretory cells that produce **mucin**. Cytoplasmic stores of mucin are not stained by conventional histochemistry and create the typical 'empty goblet' appearance.

Paneth cells are found at the base of the small intestinal crypts. They are specialized for protein synthesis and secretion and contain antibacterial proteins such as lysozyme, phospholipase A_2 and defensins. They may also have other, undefined, roles in intestinal health and disease (see Chapter 18).

Entero-endocrine cells are found predominantly near the crypt bases and produce many different enteric hormones (see Chapter 16).

Stem cells are located just above the Paneth cell zone. They retain the capacity to replenish the entire epithelium, by dividing to produce one daughter stem cell and one daughter cell that proliferates, differentiates and migrates up the crypt.

Function

Alkaline bile and **pancreatic juices** neutralize stomach acid. Powerful enzymes from the **pancreas**, which are activated in the lumen by autocatalysis and by the action of **enterokinase** released from duodenal enterocytes, support rapid and efficient **digestion**. The final stages of digestion occur in the brush border of enterocytes under the action of disaccharidases and peptidases. **Bile salts** emulsify fatty foods, allowing digestive enzymes to act more efficiently. **Transport proteins** in the apical membrane actively **absorb** sugars, amino acids and electrolytes into the enterocyte. Fatty acids and cholesterol enter by direct diffusion across the lipid membrane, are re-esterified intracellularly, complexed with apolipoproteins to form chylomicrons and released at the basolateral surface. The jejunum and ileum constitute the major digestive surfaces of the intestine, but **iron and calcium** in particular are preferentially absorbed in the duodenum (see Chapters 19–21).

The small intestine is relatively free from resident bacteria and an **antimicrobial environment** is maintained by the action of gastric acid and antibacterial substances produced by Brunner's glands and Paneth cells. Biliary epithelial cells and enterocytes transport secretory dimeric immunoglobulin A (**sIgA**) into the lumen, which may also contribute to antimicrobial defence in the small intestine (see Chapter 18).

Entero-endocrine cells in the duodenum secrete **cholecystokinin** and **secretin** in response to food, stimulating gallbladder contraction and pancreatic secretion, and inhibiting gastric **motility**. Thus, the duodenum participates in neuro-endocrine coordination of gastrointestinal function (see Chapter 16).

Common disorders

Duodenal disorders may cause epigastric **pain, diarrhoea, malabsorption, loss of weight** and **nutritional deficiencies**. Bleeding ulcers may cause **anaemia, haematemesis** and **melaena**, the characteristic black tarry appearance of stool caused by partially digested blood.

Cancer of the duodenum is extremely rare, while **peptic ulcer** and **coeliac disease** are common (see Chapters 31 & 35).

Giardia lamblia is a protozoal pathogen that causes traveller's diarrhoea, by adhering to and damaging the duodenal and jejunal epithelium, resulting in flatulence, diarrhoea and malabsorption (see Chapter 32).

7 Pancreas

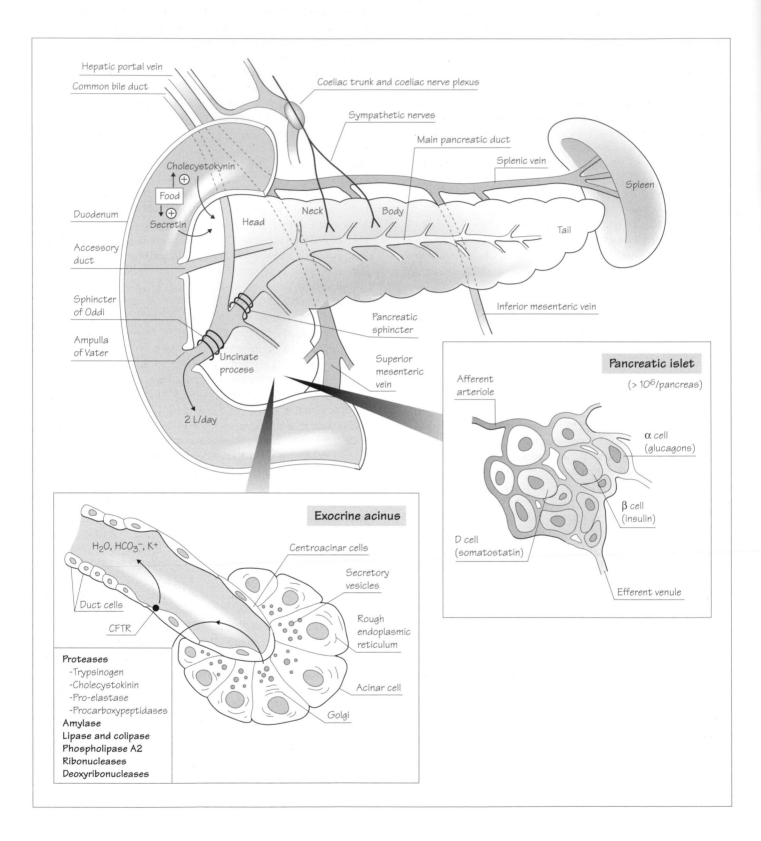

Cholecystokynin

Food

Secretin

Hepatic portal vein
Common bile duct
Coeliac trunk and coeliac nerve plexus
Sympathetic nerves
Main pancreatic duct
Splenic vein
Spleen
Duodenum
Head
Neck
Body
Tail
Accessory duct
Sphincter of Oddi
Ampulla of Vater
Uncinate process
Pancreatic sphincter
Inferior mesenteric vein
Superior mesenteric vein
2 L/day

Pancreatic islet
(> 10^6/pancreas)

Afferent arteriole
α cell (glucagons)
β cell (insulin)
D cell (somatostatin)
Efferent venule

Exocrine acinus

H_2O, HCO_3^-, K^+

Centroacinar cells
Secretory vesicles
Rough endoplasmic reticulum
Acinar cell
Golgi
Duct cells
CFTR

Proteases
- Trypsinogen
- Cholecystokinin
- Pro-elastase
- Procarboxypeptidases

Amylase
Lipase and colipase
Phospholipase A2
Ribonucleases
Deoxyribonucleases

The pancreas is critically important for intestinal digestion. It is a large **exocrine** gland, synthesizing and secreting the great majority of digestive enzymes into the intestine. It also contains important **endocrine** tissue producing insulin and glucagons, thus also regulating nutrition and gastrointestinal function globally.

Structure

The pancreas lies transversely on the posterior abdominal wall and is covered by **peritoneum**. The **head** lies to the right, adjacent to the duodenum, and the **body** and **tail** extend across the epigastrium to the spleen. The **splenic vein** runs along the superior border of the pancreas and loops of intestine are related to it anteriorly.

Branches of the **coeliac** and superior mesenteric arteries supply the gland and venous blood drains into the **hepatic portal vein**, supplying the liver with hormone- and growth factor-laden blood from the pancreas.

The **vagus** nerve and splanchnic **sympathetic nerves** innervate the pancreas. Sensory nerves are routed through the **coeliac ganglion** and pancreatic pain may be relieved by its surgical removal or destruction.

The main pancreatic **duct** extends along the length of the gland and a smaller accessory duct drains the superior part of the head and may open separately into the duodenum. The main duct joins the **common bile duct** before opening into the duodenum through the **ampulla of Vater**. Smaller pancreatic ducts drain into the main duct, forming a 'fishbone' pattern. Exocrine pancreatic tissue is arranged in **lobules** composed of the functional units, **acini**, which secrete pancreatic enzymes and fluid into the ducts.

Microscopically, pancreatic cells are arranged in **spherical acini**, with their secretory or apical surface towards the centre and the basolateral surface resting on a basement membrane. Ductules drain each acinus and coalesce to form larger ducts that eventually drain into the main pancreatic duct, carrying digestive juices to the duodenum. Pancreatic acinar cells are highly specialized for protein synthesis and secretion. They have a pyramidal cross-section, with prominent basal rough **endoplasmic reticulum**, where protein synthesis occurs, extensive **golgi** apparatus and apical secretory (**zymogen**) granules.

Over 10^6 endocrine pancreatic **islets** are scattered throughout the pancreas and are supplied with a rich capillary network of blood vessels. They are not connected by ducts to the exocrine pancreas, but secrete directly into the bloodstream. The principle cells in these islets are β **cells**, which secrete insulin, α **cells**, that secrete glucagon, and **D cells**, which synthesize somatostatin.

Function

The pancreas is a powerful producer of **digestive enzymes**. These are synthesized and stored as inactive precursors or **pro-enzymes**, to avoid autodigestion of the enzyme-producing cells and the pancreatic ducts. Pancreatic enzymes include:

- trypsinogen;
- chymotrypsinogen;
- procarboxypeptidases A and B;
- pro-elastase;
- phospholipase A;
- pancreatic lipase (and colipase);
- pancreatic amylase;
- ribonucleases;
- deoxyribonucleases.

Pancreatic secretion is stimulated by hormonal signals, particularly **cholecystokinin**, which is released when food enters the duodenum. **Secretin** enhances the effect of cholecystokinin.

The pancreas secretes about **2 L/day** of a **bicarbonate-rich alkaline** fluid that helps to neutralize stomach acid and provides optimal conditions for digestion by pancreatic enzymes. Centroacinar and duct cells secrete most of the fluid and alkali, by exchanging HCO_3^- for Cl^- ions, using the cystic fibrosis transmembrane regulator (**CFTR**) protein. Pancreatic insufficiency therefore occurs in cystic fibrosis, where an abnormal *CFTR* gene is inherited.

Pancreatic islets are the only source of **insulin and glucagon**, which are produced by pancreatic β and α cells, respectively. Insulin secretion is stimulated mainly by increased blood glucose, while glucagon secretion is stimulated by hypoglycaemia. Hormones, such as adrenaline, have additional modulatory effects on pancreatic islet secretion and islets also produce hormones, such as **somatostatin**, which modifies entero-endocrine function locally and throughout the gastrointestinal tract (see Chapter 16).

Common disorders

Pancreatic diseases may remain entirely **asymptomatic** until they are far advanced. They may cause **abdominal pain**, felt in the epigastrium and radiating to the back. Damage to the common pancreatic and bile ducts may cause **jaundice** and pancreatic exocrine insufficiency may result in **malabsorption** of food, causing **diarrhoea**, **steatorrhoea** (fat-rich stools), **weight loss** and **nutritional deficiencies**. Islet damage can cause **diabetes mellitus**.

Acute pancreatitis is a serious, potentially life-threatening illness. The most common causes are excess alcohol ingestion and passage of gallstones through the ampulla of Vater (see Chapter 40). Less frequent causes include various drugs, abdominal trauma and viral infection. The inflamed pancreas releases enzymes into the circulation and acute pancreatitis is a systemic illness, affecting the whole body. Pancreatic lipases release fatty acids that interact with calcium to form insoluble calcium-fatty acyl salts, potentially lowering the concentration of calcium in the circulation to dangerous levels. A dramatic rise in the serum **lipase or amylase level** helps to diagnose acute pancreatitis.

Chronic pancreatitis may follow repeated bouts of acute pancreatitis. The main symptoms are abdominal pain and malabsorption due to failure of the exocrine pancreas. Patients may also develop endocrine pancreatic insufficiency (see Chapter 40).

Pancreatic **adenocarcinoma** is a leading cause of cancer-related death and often becomes symptomatic only at an advanced stage, when the tumour has become inoperable. **Neuro-endocrine tumours**, which arise from enteric endocrine cells, are often located in the pancreas, although they may also arise from other parts of the gastrointestinal tract. They are generally less aggressive than adenocarcinoma, but may cause symptoms due to their secretion of gut hormones. Gastrin-producing tumours (**gastrinomas**) cause excess gastric acid secretion and peptic ulceration (**Zollinger–Ellison syndrome**). Tumours may also secrete insulin, glucagon and other hormones (see Chapters 16 & 38).

8 Liver

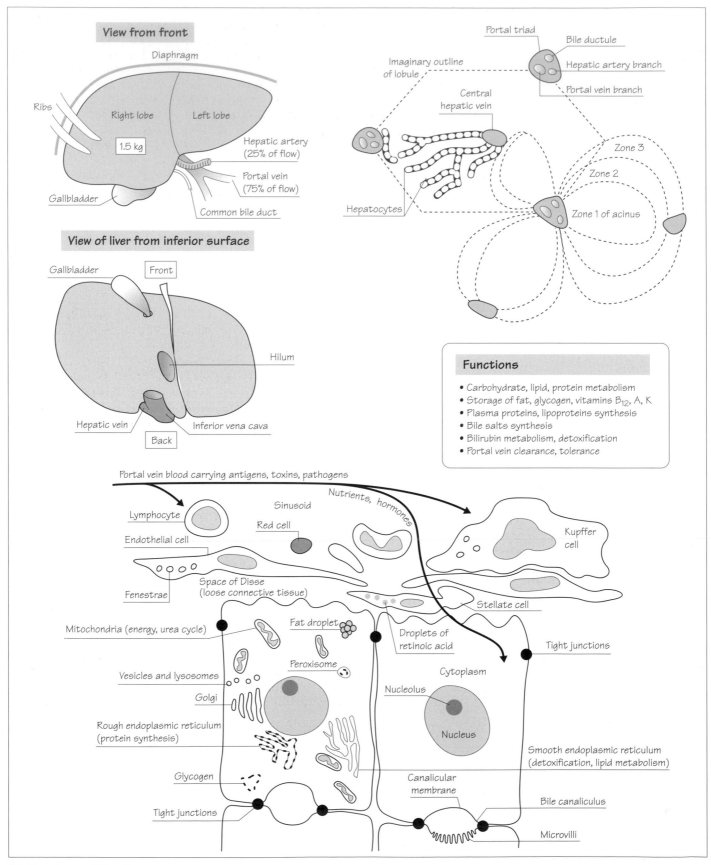

View from front

Diaphragm

Ribs

Right lobe   Left lobe

1.5 kg

Gallbladder

Hepatic artery (25% of flow)

Portal vein (75% of flow)

Common bile duct

View of liver from inferior surface

Gallbladder   Front

Hilum

Hepatic vein   Inferior vena cava

Back

Portal triad

Bile ductule

Hepatic artery branch

Imaginary outline of lobule

Portal vein branch

Central hepatic vein

Zone 3

Zone 2

Zone 1 of acinus

Hepatocytes

Functions

- Carbohydrate, lipid, protein metabolism
- Storage of fat, glycogen, vitamins B_{12}, A, K
- Plasma proteins, lipoproteins synthesis
- Bile salts synthesis
- Bilirubin metabolism, detoxification
- Portal vein clearance, tolerance

Portal vein blood carrying antigens, toxins, pathogens

Nutrients, hormones

Lymphocyte

Sinusoid

Red cell

Kupffer cell

Endothelial cell

Space of Disse (loose connective tissue)

Fenestrae

Stellate cell

Mitochondria (energy, urea cycle)

Fat droplet

Droplets of retinoic acid

Tight junctions

Vesicles and lysosomes

Peroxisome

Cytoplasm

Nucleolus

Golgi

Rough endoplasmic reticulum (protein synthesis)

Nucleus

Smooth endoplasmic reticulum (detoxification, lipid metabolism)

Glycogen

Canalicular membrane

Tight junctions

Bile canaliculus

Microvilli

The liver is the largest solid organ in the body, weighing **1.5 kg** in a 70-kg adult. It develops from the embryonic foregut endoderm and is an integral part of the gastrointestinal system. It performs vital metabolic, synthetic, secretory and excretory roles, and life cannot be sustained for more than a few hours without the liver.

Structure

The liver lies in the **right upper quadrant** of the abdomen, directly under the right hemidiaphragm, protected by the lower ribs. It crosses the mid-line, where the falciform ligament traverses it, separating the left **lobe** from the right. The liver can be divided into nine **functional segments** that can be identified surgically, based on vascular supply and biliary drainage.

On the inferior surface, in the mid-line, the portal vein and hepatic artery enter and common bile duct and lymphatic channels leave the **hilum** of the liver. These structures divide into major right and left branches within the liver. The **inferior vena cava** traverses the liver posteriorly, where the main **hepatic vein** joins it.

The **gallbladder** lies under the liver to the right of the mid-line and is connected to the common bile duct by the **cystic duct**. The hepatic flexure of the colon lies to the right of the gallbladder. The liver parenchyma is enclosed in a tough fibrous **capsule**, which is mostly covered by **peritoneum**, apart from the **bare area** under the dome of the diaphragm.

The **hepatic artery**, arising from the **coeliac trunk** delivers arterial blood to the liver, although 75% of the hepatic blood flow arrives via the **portal vein**, which drains the spleen, pancreas and intestines. Venous drainage is via the **hepatic vein**.

Microscopically the liver **parenchyma** is homogeneous, with repetition of the same basic organization throughout. **Hepatocytes** form **three-dimensional cords and plates** in the liver. These are separated by **sinusoids** through which blood flows slowly. There are two main ways of conceptualizing the microscopic arrangement. In the **lobular model**, the hepatic venule is at the centre, with portal vein branches at three corners of a six-sided lobule. In the **acinar model**, the portal vein and hepatic artery branches and bile ductules are at the centre in the **portal triads**, with three zones (1, 2 and 3) defined by their distance from the centre.

The walls of adjacent hepatocytes form **bile canaliculi**. Specialized **biliary epithelial cells** line small bile ductules, larger ducts and the gallbladder.

Hepatic **stellate cells**, also known as Ito cells or fat cells because they contain prominent droplets of fat and **retinoic acid** (a vitamin A derivative), are situated deep to the sinusoidal endothelium. They elaborate the connective tissue matrix of the liver and respond to injury by causing **fibrosis**.

Endothelial cells line the sinusoids. They rest on a loose connective tissue matrix, known as the **space of Disse**, and are discontinuous. They also contain gaps or **fenestrae**, which may allow molecules, particles and even cells to easily penetrate the parenchyma from the sinusoids.

Within sinusoids, resident macrophages called **Kupffer cells** interact with particles and cells. Numerous lymphoid cells are present, including special subsets of **lymphocytes** and **dendritic cells**. Their function is unknown, although they probably contribute to special immunological properties of the liver (see Chapter 18).

Hepatocytes are large, **cuboidal** cells with a central nucleus that is occasionally tetraploid. They are functionally **polarized**, with **sinusoidal** and **canalicular** poles. **Tight junctions** and desmosomes seal off the canalicular membranes, across which hepatocytes secrete the constituents of **bile**. **Microvilli** help to increase the cell surface area.

Hepatocytes are extremely metabolically active and contain many **intracellular organelles**. There is extensive **smooth endoplasmic reticulum** for lipid and cholesterol synthesis and **rough endoplasmic reticulum** for protein synthesis. There are many **mitochondria** in which metabolic reactions, such as the Krebs cycle, occur and where chemical energy is generated. There are **lysosomes**, **peroxisomes** and endocytic vesicles supporting digestive functions, and **storage vacuoles**, **glycogen granules** and **fat droplets**.

Function

The liver's complex functions have not yet been reproduced artificially. They include:

- Regulating **homeostasis** of carbohydrate, lipid and amino acid metabolism.
- **Storing nutrients** such as glycogen, fats and vitamins B_{12}, A and K.
- Producing and secreting **plasma proteins** and lipoproteins, including clotting factors and acute phase proteins.
- Synthesizing and secreting **bile salts** for lipid digestion.
- **Detoxifying** and **excreting** bilirubin, other endogenous waste products and exogenous metal ions, drugs and toxins (**xenobiotics**).
- **Clearing** toxins and infective agents from the **portal venous** blood whilst maintaining systemic immune **tolerance** to antigens in the portal circulation.

In addition, hepatocytes retain the capacity to **proliferate**, so that the liver can **regenerate** dramatically after injury.

Common disorders

Liver disorders can cause many symptoms and signs, ranging from vague **malaise** to fulminant liver failure, with disordered **coagulation** and **coma**. Typical features include **jaundice**, **fatigue**, **loss of appetite** and **pain** in the right upper quadrant of the abdomen. Because of the great reserve capacity of the liver, extensive damage may remain **asymptomatic**.

Viral hepatitis is common throughout the world. **Liver abscesses**, caused by amoebae, bacteria and parasites, are common in some parts of the world. **Drugs and toxins**, including medications, also commonly affect the liver and the most important of these is **alcohol**. Chronic damage may cause scarring and lead to **cirrhosis**. Overwhelming liver damage, either acutely or chronically, causes **liver failure**. Although primary liver cancer is rare, **metastatic cancers** are common (see Chapters 33, 38, 41 & 42).

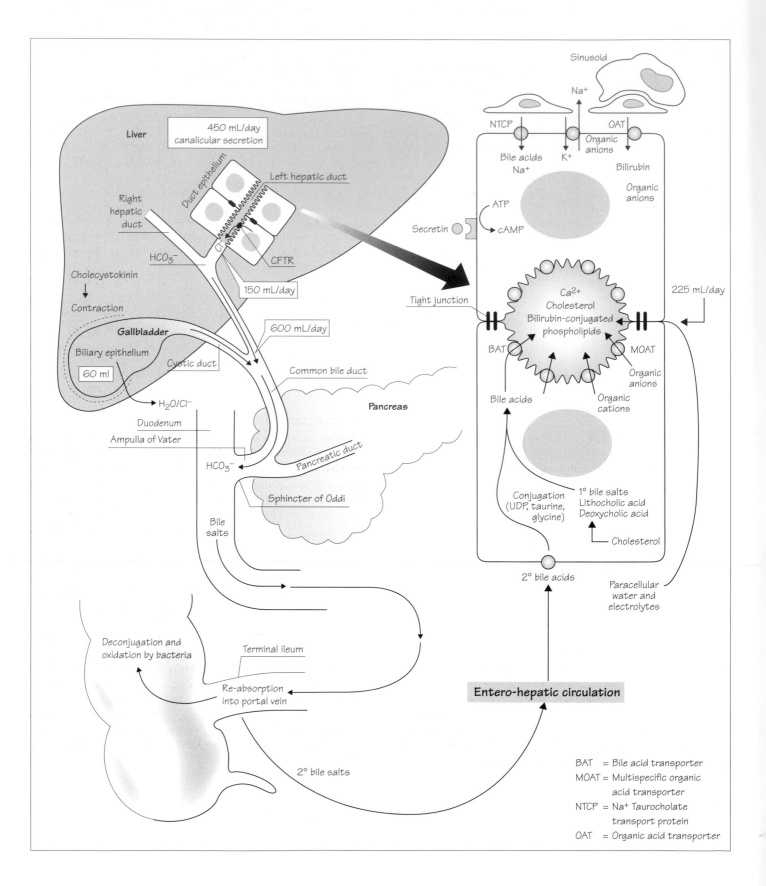

Bile is formed by hepatocytes and modified by the specialized biliary epithelium. It is an exocrine secretion necessary for digestion, an excretion product for removal of toxins and metabolic waste and a part of the host defence system.

Structure

Macroscopically, the intrahepatic **bile ducts**, common hepatic duct, cystic duct, **gallbladder** and common bile duct constitute the biliary system.

The gallbladder is a pouch-like structure with a thin **fibromuscular** wall located under the anterior edge of the liver. Its epithelium is thrown up in complex **fronds**, increasing the surface area. The **neck** of the gallbladder leads to the **cystic duct**, which joins the common hepatic duct, formed from the union of the right and left intrahepatic ducts, to form the **common bile duct**, which leaves the liver at the hilum. The common bile duct lies adjacent to the hepatic artery and portal vein and joins the main **pancreatic duct** before entering the duodenum through the **ampulla of Vater**, which is kept closed by the **sphincter of Oddi**.

The biliary epithelium lining the major ducts and the gallbladder is composed of a single layer of **columnar** or **cuboidal cells** resting on a basement membrane. It can **secrete** Cl^- and water and in the gallbladder the same cells **absorb** water, to concentrate bile.

The biliary **canaliculus** is the primary site of bile production. It is a channel formed from apposed surfaces of adjacent **hepatocytes**. Tight junctions separate the canalicular membrane from the basolateral surface of the hepatocyte, allowing transport proteins to create and maintain concentration gradients. As biliary canaliculi converge and enlarge, specialized biliary epithelial cells replace hepatocytes.

Function

Each day, **600 mL** of thick, mucoid, alkaline bile is produced. Its main constituents are:

- **primary bile acids**: cholic and chenodeoxycholic acid;
- **secondary bile acids**: deoxycholic and lithocholic acid;
- **phospholipids**;
- **cholesterol**;
- **bilirubin**;
- conjugated drugs and endogenous **waste products**;
- **electrolytes**: Na^+, Cl^-, HCO_3^- and trace metals, such as copper;
- secretory dimeric immunoglobulin A (**sIgA**) and other antibacterial proteins;
- **mucin** glycoproteins.

Transporter proteins on the basolateral surface of the hepatocyte, such as the organic acid transport (**OAT**) protein, facilitate uptake of substances such as bilirubin and bile salts from the circulation. Transporters in the canalicular membrane then secrete compounds from the hepatocyte into bile. Important canalicular transporters include the bile acid transporter (**BAT**) and the multispecific organic anion transporter (**MOAT**). Specific transporters help to excrete potential toxins; for example, excess **copper** is excreted by an adenosine triphosphate (ATP) -dependent copper transporter that is defective in **Wilson's disease**, causing accumulation of copper in the brain and liver.

Active secretion of bile acids, electrolytes and organic compounds draws **water** with it and bile flow is encouraged by coordinated contraction of **cytoskeletal proteins** adjacent to the canalicular membrane. The canaliculi secrete 450 mL/day and bile ducts add 150 mL/day.

About 60 mL of bile is stored in the gallbladder. Cholesterol is a major insoluble constituent of bile and it is stabilized by incorporation into **mixed micelles**, formed by bile salts and phospholipids.

Abnormal bile may be formed if hepatocytes are overloaded with one or other component; for example, **haemolysis** results in overproduction of bilirubin, which may crystallize to form gallstones.

Cholecystokinin is released from the duodenum when food arrives in it, stimulating contraction of the gallbladder and relaxation of the sphincter of Oddi, thus delivering bile to the duodenum just when it is needed.

Bile promotes the **digestion** and absorption of fats and fat-soluble vitamins in several ways. The alkaline bile promotes **emulsification** of fats, which allows greater access to digestive enzymes, and **bile acids**, cholesterol and phospholipids form **mixed micelles**, into which digested fatty acids and other lipids are incorporated. The **alkaline pH** is also optimal for pancreatic lipases.

Primary bile acids are synthesized in the liver from **cholesterol** and 95% of the secreted bile acids are reabsorbed in the terminal ileum and carried into the portal venous circulation. These **secondary bile acids**, which have been metabolized by bacteria in the intestine, are taken up by hepatocytes and resecreted into the bile. This constitutes the **enterohepatic circulation** (see Chapter 24).

Bile is the main pathway for **excretion** of hydrophobic wastes such as bilirubin.

Common disorders

Jaundice, caused by accumulation of bilirubin, is the classic symptom of biliary disease. Interrupting bile flow to the intestine causes **pale stool** and **dark urine** as bilirubin is excreted via the urine. **Itching** is caused by accumulation of pruritogenic substances that are normally excreted in bile. Longstanding obstruction interferes with fat absorption and may cause **steatorrhoea**, **weight loss** and **nutritional deficiency**. Obstruction and inflammation of the biliary tract can cause **pain**, **fever** and **malaise** (see Chapters 33 & 40).

Damage to hepatocytes, for example by **viral hepatitis**, may inhibit bile secretion, by decreasing ATP levels, interfering with transporter function and damaging cytoskeletal proteins. This causes **intrahepatic cholestasis**, with no macroscopic blockage to the biliary system. Certain drugs can produce a similar effect (see Chapter 41).

Autoimmune damage to intrahepatic bile ducts, in **primary biliary cirrhosis (PBC)**, causes progressive jaundice and liver damage.

Gallstones are very common and may remain asymptomatic. They form when constituents, such as cholesterol or bile pigments, that are partially soluble, reach supersaturated concentrations and crystallize around a **nidus**, such as a stray bacterial cell. They can cause **cholecystitis** in the gallbladder and **cholangitis** or **pancreatitis** when they lodge in the bile ducts, causing obstruction and superadded infection (see Chapter 40).

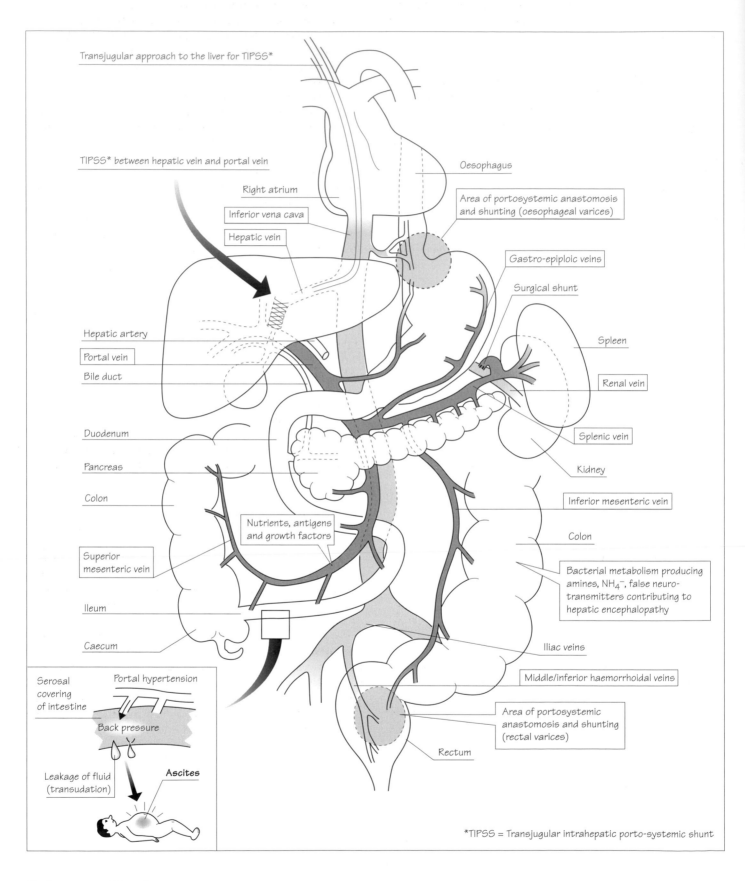

Transjugular approach to the liver for TIPSS*

TIPSS* between hepatic vein and portal vein

Right atrium

Inferior vena cava

Hepatic vein

Oesophagus

Area of portosystemic anastomosis and shunting (oesophageal varices)

Gastro-epiploic veins

Surgical shunt

Hepatic artery

Portal vein

Bile duct

Spleen

Renal vein

Splenic vein

Kidney

Duodenum

Pancreas

Colon

Inferior mesenteric vein

Colon

Nutrients, antigens and growth factors

Superior mesenteric vein

Bacterial metabolism producing amines, NH_4^-, false neuro-transmitters contributing to hepatic encephalopathy

Ileum

Caecum

Iliac veins

Middle/inferior haemorrhoidal veins

Serosal covering of intestine

Portal hypertension

Back pressure

Leakage of fluid (transudation)

Ascites

Area of portosystemic anastomosis and shunting (rectal varices)

Rectum

*TIPSS = Transjugular intrahepatic porto-systemic shunt

The liver receives 25% of the cardiac output, of which 75% arrives via the portal vein, which drains the spleen, pancreas and gastrointestinal tract from stomach to colon. Thus, all the blood from these organs normally traverses the liver before it enters the systemic circulation. This arrangement serves many important functions.

Structure

The portal vein is formed from the confluence of the **splenic vein**, which drains the stomach, pancreas and spleen, and the **superior mesenteric vein**, which drains the entire small intestine and most of the large intestine. The **inferior mesenteric vein**, which drains the rest of the large intestine, joins the splenic vein. The portal vein enters the liver at the **hilum**, alongside the hepatic artery and common bile duct.

Within the liver the portal vein divides, first into left and right main branches and then further, so that small branches supply each **acinus** or **lobule**. These small branches lie in **portal triads**, with branches of the hepatic artery and bile ducts, surrounded by a small amount of connective tissue. Portal venous blood flows slowly through the **hepatic sinusoids** and exits the liver through terminal hepatic venules, which join to form the **hepatic veins**, rejoining the systemic circulation at the inferior vena cava (see Chapter 8).

Importantly, the venous drainage of the **oesophagus** and lower **rectum** goes directly into the systemic circulation, bypassing the portal venous system and the liver. When portal venous flow is obstructed, **collaterals** develop in these (and other) areas, joining portal and systemic circulations, causing **portosystemic shunting**. Increased flow causes the collateral veins to dilate and enlarge, forming **varices**, which can bleed. Furthermore, when blood is diverted away from the portal circulation, it enters the systemic circulation directly, without first being detoxified by the liver.

Function

Nutrients and **hormones** from the pancreas and intestine are carried by the portal vein to the liver, enabling it to regulate nutrition and metabolism. Hepatocytes cannot survive without the portal circulation, even if total blood flow is maintained from the systemic arterial circulation. This is probably due its need for growth factors, including **insulin**, derived from the intestines and pancreas.

The liver removes **toxins** that are ingested with food and produced by **bacterial metabolism** in the intestine. Toxic products of bacterial metabolism include amino acids that mimic neurotransmitters, such as glutamine and γ-amino butyric acid (GABA), and ammonia, which interfere with mental function, contributing to **hepatic encephalopathy**.

Medicines absorbed from the intestine first encounter the liver, where they can be efficiently metabolized. This '**first-pass metabolism**' is so efficient for some drugs that the oral dose has to be increased or an alternative route of administration, for example, sublingual or parenteral, substituted. Some drugs are designed for clearance by the liver, preserving the local therapeutic effect in the intestine, while the first-pass metabolism removes the drug from the systemic circulation, reducing side-effects. The synthetic glucocorticoid **budesonide**, which is used to treat inflammatory bowel disease, is an example.

Microorganisms inevitably cross the intestinal epithelium and enter the bloodstream (**bacterial translocation**). **Kupffer cells** in the hepatic sinusoids normally clear them effectively. Patients with chronic liver disease and portal hypertension are therefore at increased risk of bacterial infection.

The body recognizes that **food antigens** are usually harmless, and they generally do not elicit an immune response, a phenomenon called **oral tolerance**. The liver contributes to this, and antigens injected into the portal vein also induce tolerance.

Portal hypertension

Liver cirrhosis is the commonest cause of portal hypertension but it may also occur when the liver is congested in **chronic heart failure** or with **portal vein thrombosis**, for example following trauma or infection. Portal hypertension causes **splenomegaly** and **ascites**. Portosystemic shunting causes **varices** to form and, particularly if there is severe underlying liver disease, it causes hepatic **encephalopathy**.

Splenomegaly may cause hypersplenism and thrombocytopenia as platelets are trapped in the enlarged spleen.

Ascites is the accumulation of fluid in the peritoneal space. Portal hypertension increases hydrostatic pressure in intestinal and mesenteric capillaries, causing fluid leakage. The protein concentration of this ascitic fluid is low (**transudate**) and it lacks antibacterial factors, such as **complement**, so that it is prone to becoming infected, resulting in **spontaneous bacterial peritonitis**.

Varices may form in the oesophagus and gastric fundus, around the splenic hilum, at the umbilicus, in the rectum and in scar tissue and adhesions created by abdominal surgery. They are prone to damage and may **rupture**, causing massive, life-threatening **gastrointestinal haemorrhage**. This usually causes **haematemesis**, **melaena** or **haematochesia** (rectal bleeding).

Encephalopathy causes disturbances of **memory**, a characteristic flapping tremor of the hands (**asterixis**), clumsiness and an inability to draw simple shapes (**constructional apraxia**), and **drowsiness**, which can progress to **coma**. Encephalopathy is caused by **shunting** of toxins to the systemic circulation and is worse when the capacity of the **liver** to inactivate toxins is reduced. It is also aggravated by **gastrointestinal haemorrhage**, as blood protein is digested, releasing excess amino acids that are broken down to release **ammonia**, which contributes to the encephalopathy.

Portal pressure can be reduced by creating an artificial portosystemic shunt or with drugs such as β-blockers. **Surgical shunts** can connect the portal vein to the inferior vena cava, or a flexible metal stent can be placed within the liver, via the jugular vein, under radiological guidance. This is called a transjugular intrahepatic portosystemic shunt (**TIPSS**). Shunts can reduce varices and ascites, and aggravate encephalopathy.

11 Jejunum and ileum

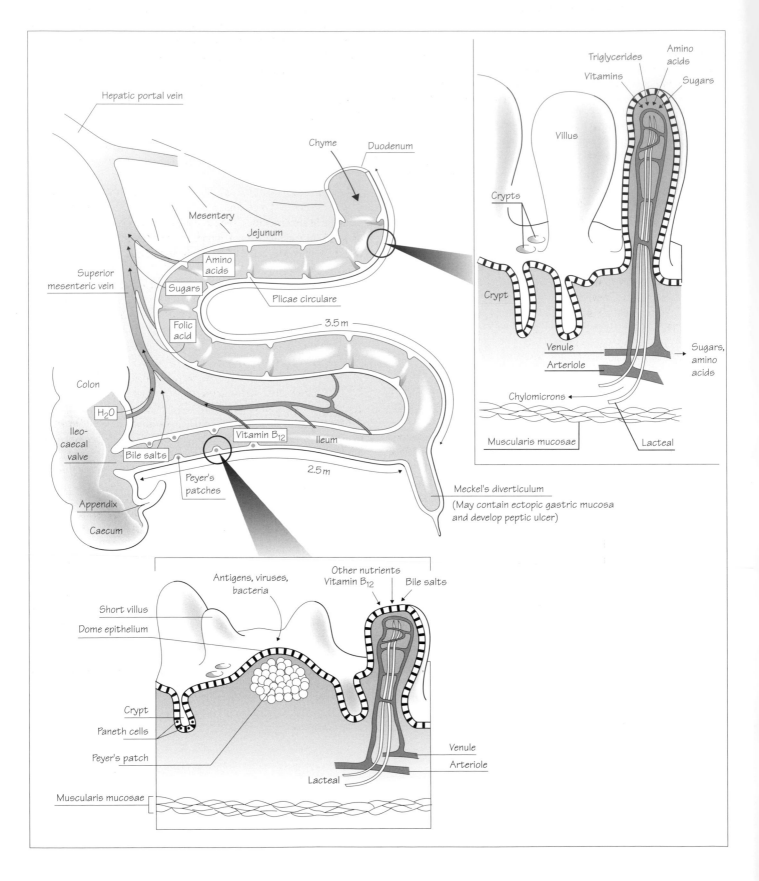

The jejunum and ileum are the main absorptive surfaces of the gastrointestinal tract. They are essential for life and intestinal failure occurs when surgery or disease leaves less than a metre of functional small intestine.

Structure

The **jejunum** begins at the junction with the duodenum at the ligament of Treitz and measures about **3.5 m**. The **ileum** comprises the most distal 2.5 m of small intestine, terminating in the caecum. A loose, redundant fold of mucosa protrudes into the caecum, forming a flap, the **ileocaecal valve**, which prevents reflux of caecal contents into the terminal ileum.

The jejunum and ileum are attached to the posterior abdominal wall by a long **mesentery** that allows free movement and rotation, so that the position of loops of small intestine is highly variable.

The **blood supply** is derived from the **superior mesenteric artery**. Venous drainage is via the superior mesenteric vein into the **portal vein** and lymphatics drain into the **thoracic duct** via mesenteric lymph nodes and ascending lymphoid channels.

The **microscopic structure** of the jejunum and ileum is similar to that of the duodenum, except that Brunner's glands are absent (see Chapter 6). Jejunal villi are long, broad and leaf-shaped, while ileal villi are shorter, rounder and more blunted. Jejunal crypts are deeper than ileal crypts and contain fewer Paneth cells. Plicae circulare, which are submucosal folds, increase surface area and are most prominent in the jejunum. The size of the lumen gradually reduces distally. **Peyer's patches** are most prominent in the distal ileum.

Function

Mucosal enzymes, particularly disaccharidases and peptidases complete the digestive processes initiated by pancreatic enzymes in the lumen (see Chapter 20).

In addition, jejunal epithelial cells express specialized enzymatic pathways to process and absorb dietary **folic acid**. The terminal ileal epithelium is specialized for the digestion of **vitamin B_{12}**, which is disassociated from intrinsic factor in the terminal ileum (see Chapter 21).

Bile salts are released from mixed micelles as fats are digested and absorbed proximally and are reabsorbed in the terminal ileum through specific transport proteins. The liver then recycles bile salts through the **entero-hepatic circulation**. Specialized ileal function is therefore essential for healthy nutrition (see Chapter 24).

Approximately **1 m** of functioning small intestine must remain to allow adequate absorption of nutrients. Surgery or disease that leaves less than this causes **short-bowel syndrome** and **intestinal failure**.

There is more lymphoid tissue in the distal ileum than the jejunum and proximal intestine. This reflects a higher bacterial load and, as the terminal ileum is also particularly prone to Crohn's disease, intestinal tuberculosis and *Yersinia* infection, it may serve a more fundamental immunological function (see Chapters 18, 33 & 34).

Common disorders

Abdominal **pain**, **diarrhoea**, **flatulence**, **weight loss** and nutritio deficiencies are the main symptoms of small intestinal disorder **Obstruction** of the small intestine may be caused by disease within the intestine, or by external compression, or twisting, as in a strangulated hernia. Typical symptoms are **pain**, **anorexia** and **vomiting**.

Chronic infection with *Giardia lamblia*, and with various roundworms, hookworms and tapeworms, is a common cause of malabsorption in endemic areas. Microsporidia and cryptosporidia are particularly troublesome in immunocompromised individuals, causing intractable diarrhoea.

Salmonella typhi, the cause of **typhoid fever**, gains entry into the body through Peyer's patches, which may become acutely inflamed and can perforate.

Commensal bacteria that are normally found only in the large intestine may overgrow and accumulate in the small intestine in patients with anatomical abnormalities, such as congenital pouches and diverticulae, or surgically created blind loops, or with motility disorders. **Bacterial overgrowth** causes flatulence, abdominal pain, diarrhoea and malabsorption.

Tropical sprue is associated with chronic bacterial infection of the intestine, particularly in visitors to tropical regions, and causes malabsorption due to damage to the small intestinal mucosa. Its incidence has declined dramatically.

Neoplasia is rare and the most frequent tumours are benign or maligant neuro-endocrine tumours, lymphomas and smooth muscle tumours. In areas of high endemic gastrointestinal infection, such as the Far East, a form of small intestinal lymphoma known as immunoproliferative small intestinal disease (**IPSID**) is relatively frequent.

Meckel's diverticulum in the small intestine, at the site of attachment to the embryonic yolk sac, may contain ectopic, acid-secreting gastric mucosa that can develop peptic ulceration, causing pain and bleeding. It is the most common malformation of the small intestine, but is rarely symptomatic.

Crohn's disease can affect any part of the intestine, but in about 60% of cases it preferentially affects the terminal ileum, causing mucosal ulceration and transmural granulomatous inflammation. An inflammatory mass and fistulae between the small intestine and adjacent structures, such as the bladder, may occur. Crohn's disease of the terminal ileum has been shown to be associated with mutations in the *NOD2* gene, which may determine how monocytes and Paneth cells interact with enteric bacteria (see Chapter 34). Ileocaecal **tuberculosis** and *Yersinia enterocolitica* infection can appear clinically identical to ileal Crohn's disease.

Loops of small intestine are extremely mobile and may be caught in **hernial sacs** or in adhesions. This can cause **intestinal obstruction**, which may need to be relieved surgically.

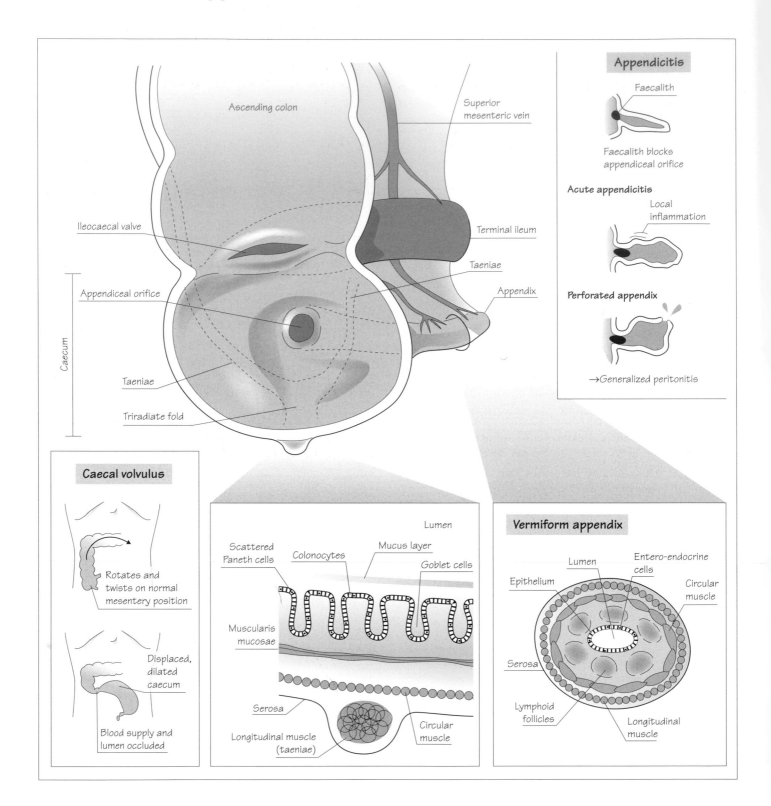

Ascending colon

Superior
mesenteric vein

Ileocaecal valve

Terminal ileum

Appendiceal orifice

Taeniae

Appendix

Caecum

Taeniae

Triradiate fold

Appendicitis

Faecalith

Faecalith blocks
appendiceal orifice

Acute appendicitis

Local
inflammation

Perforated appendix

→Generalized peritonitis

Caecal volvulus

Rotates and
twists on normal
mesentery position

Displaced,
dilated
caecum

Blood supply and
lumen occluded

Lumen

Scattered
Paneth cells

Colonocytes

Mucus layer

Goblet cells

Muscularis
mucosae

Serosa

Longitudinal muscle
(taeniae)

Circular
muscle

Vermiform appendix

Lumen

Entero-endocrine
cells

Epithelium

Circular
muscle

Serosa

Lymphoid
follicles

Longitudinal
muscle

The caecum is the most proximal part of the large intestine, into which the ileum opens. The appendix is a blind-ended tube protruding from the caecum.

Structure

The caecum and appendix lie in the right iliac fossa. The **ileocaecal valve**, protruding into the lumen of the large intestine, marks the upper border of the caecum, which extends down to form a bowl-shaped cavity. The appendix lies in the distal portion of the caecum and is connected to it by a slit-like opening.

The blood supply is derived from branches of the **superior mesenteric artery** and drains via the **superior mesenteric vein** into the portal vein. Lymphatics drain into the thoracic duct via mesenteric lymph nodes and ascending lymphoid channels.

The caecum and appendix are connected to the posterior abdominal wall on a variable length of **mesentery**, which generally fixes the caecum to the posterior abdominal wall and leaves the appendix more freely mobile.

The caecal walls are relatively thin and the longitudinal muscle layer is gathered into three cords, or **taeniae**, which meet at the apex of the caecum, forming a **triradiate fold** that can be seen during colonoscopy.

The microscopic structure of the caecum is typical of the large intestinal epithelium, with **no villi** and deep **crypts** (see Chapter 13). The epithelial cells are mainly mature enterocytes and **goblet cells** with scattered entero-endocrine and Paneth cells.

The epithelium of the appendix may be disrupted and ulcerated, exposing the extensive **lymphoid tissue** in the mucosa and submucosa. Entero-endocrine cells are scattered through the epithelium.

Function

The caecum and appendix apparently have no special function in humans, although in other species they are well developed, containing **commensal bacteria** that metabolize complex plant carbohydrates, particularly cellulose, that cannot be digested by mammalian enzymes.

Lymphoid tissue in the appendix may somehow contribute to **immune regulation**; for example, the incidence of **ulcerative colitis** is reduced in people who have had an **appendicectomy**.

Common disorders

Appendicitis results from obstruction of the appendiceal lumen, causing infection and inflammation. An obstructing **faecalith** is often seen when surgery is performed for appendicitis. Initially, appendicitis causes **peri-umbilical pain**, nausea and vomiting. This is because **visceral nerves** from mid-gut structures refer pain to the peri-umbilical area and stimulate the **vomiting centre**. As inflammation progresses, reaching the outside of the appendix, from the parietal peritoneum nerve fibres carry precise spatial information to the **somatosensory** cortex and pain is localized to the **right iliac fossa**, overlying the inflamed appendix. Untreated, appendicitis may progress to form an appendiceal **abscess** or rupture into the peritoneal cavity, causing **peritonitis**.

Bacterial translocation into the veins draining the appendix may travel in the portal vein to the liver, where they may cause **liver abscess** (see Chapter 33).

Carcinoid tumours occur frequently in the appendix, where they may remain asymptomatic.

The thin-walled caecum is prone to **perforation**, for example, due to intestinal obstruction or in severe colitis (toxic dilatation) (see Chapter 34).

Caecal volvulus occurs when the caecum twists on its own mesentery, obstructing the lumen and the blood supply, ultimately causing necrosis and perforation.

Tuberculosis and **Crohn's disease** can affect the caecum, as can **colorectal cancer**. Unfortunately, caecal tumours can remain asymptomatic for a long time and so may only be detected at a late stage.

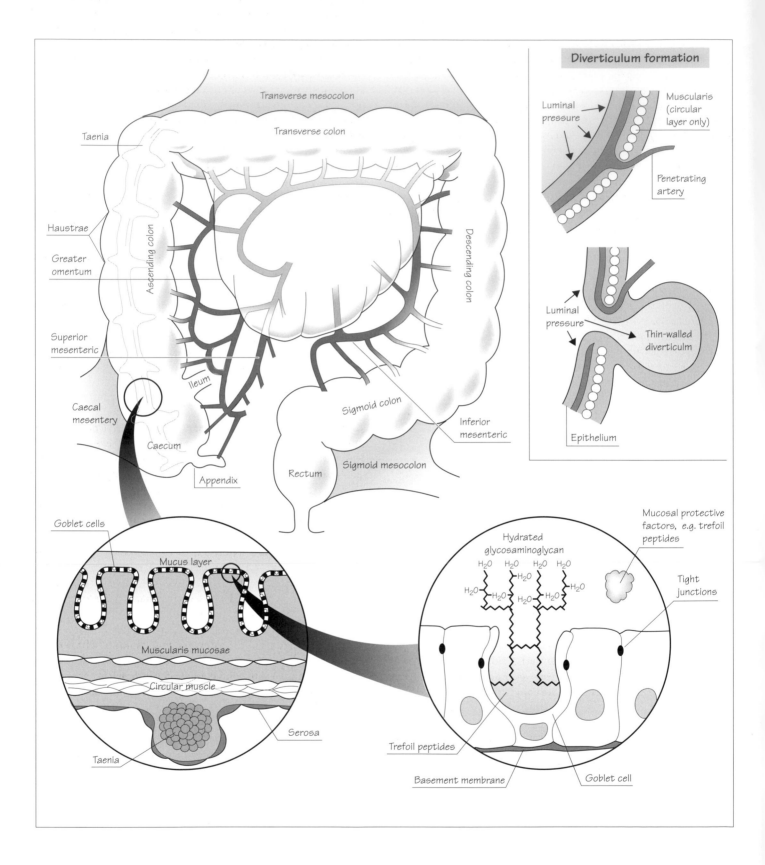

The colon comprises most of the large intestine, is about 1.5 m long and is not essential for life.

Structure

The colon is divided into four parts. The **ascending** colon begins at the top of the caecum and ascends in the right flank to the inferior surface of the liver, where it turns sharply to the left—the **hepatic flexure**. This is the start of the **transverse** colon, which forms a lax arch of variable length from right to left. It ends at the spleen, turning sharply downwards and backwards, forming the **splenic flexure** and joining the **descending** colon, which descends along the left flank to the pelvic rim. Here it joins the **sigmoid** colon, which is fixed at its upper end, and at its lower end where it joins the **rectum**. In between, it curves over the pelvic brim, suspended on a length of mesentery.

The ascending and descending colon are largely **retroperitoneal**, while the transverse colon is suspended on a short mesentery attached to the posterior abdominal wall.

The **greater omentum** is a sheet of mesentery covered with peritoneal epithelium and filled with fatty, loose connective tissue. It is suspended from the lower border of the transverse colon, forming an intra-abdominal apron-like structure and is a site of **fat storage**, accounting for some of the abdominal girth of obese middle-aged people.

The **superior mesenteric** artery supplies the ascending colon and the proximal transverse colon, and the **inferior mesenteric artery** supplies the remainder of the colon. Venous drainage is via the **superior** and **inferior mesenteric veins** into the **hepatic portal vein**.

The wall of the colon reflects the general organization of the intestinal tract, although the external longitudinal muscle is discontinuous. The layers are, from the outside in:

* serosa;
* longitudinal muscle layer (taenia);
* circular muscle layer;
* submucosa;
* muscularis mucosae;
* mucosal layer comprising the lamina propria and a simple columnar epithelial lining.

The longitudinal muscle layer is collected into three bands or **taeniae**. These are in constant tonic contraction, shortening the colon and producing characteristic saccular bulges (**haustrae**).

The lamina propria contains fibroblasts, lymphocytes and other leucocytes, entero-chromaffin cells, nerve cell processes and blood vessels, but lacks lymphatic vessels, which is why lymphatic invasion occurs relatively late in colon cancer.

The colonic epithelium lacks villi and has numerous **crypts** that open onto the surface. It is lined by a single layer of columnar epithelial cells (**colonocytes**), goblet cells and scattered entero-endocrine cells. **Stem cells** reside at the crypt bases. There are a few Paneth cells in the ascending colon, even in healthy individuals, and numbers are increased in inflammatory bowel disease (IBD).

Goblet cells produce copious amounts of **mucus** that coats the epithelium in a tough, hydrated layer, protecting it from mechanical trauma and bacterial invasion. The main constituents of mucus are polypeptide chains held together by disulphide bonds, which are heavily glycosylated (**glycosaminoglycans**). The extensive carbohydrate side chains attract water and become hydrated, forming a slippery **gel**. Goblet cells also produce **trefoil peptides**, which contribute to host defence by stimulating epithelial healing.

Blood vessels supplying the colon penetrate the circular muscle layer, creating a gap and a potential mechanical weakness. In the sigmoid colon particularly, these gaps can allow herniation of the mucosa and, with time, allow pouches or **diverticulae** to form.

Function

The major function of the colon is to **reabsorb water** from the liquid intestinal contents remaining after digestion and absorption in the jejunum and ileum. This converts the faecal stream into a semisolid mass that is then excreted. Muscular action in the colon mixes and squeezes faecal matter and propels it toward the rectum. Total colectomy is well tolerated, apart from potential fluid and electrolyte depletion that can be avoided by ingesting extra salt and water.

The colon contains 10^{12} **bacteria/g** of its content, which are normal commensals. There are about **500 different species** of bacteria, including lactobacilli, bifidobacteriae, bacteroides and enterobacteriacae. Most colonic bacteria are **anaerobes**. Some are **potential pathogens**, such as the clostridial species and *Escherichia coli*, which can acquire virulence factors via plasmids and bacteriophages. The balance of species in the commensal flora probably helps to maintain health and, conversely, alterations in this balance may contribute to illness (see Chapters 32–34).

Common disorders

Abdominal pain, **altered bowel habit** (constipation or diarrhoea) and **flatulence** are common symptoms arising from colonic disorders. Bleeding may cause **anaemia** or may be detected as visible blood in the stool (**haematochesia**), or by special testing for **faecal occult blood** (see Chapter 43).

Colon and rectal cancer (**colorectal cancer**) is the second most common cause of cancer-related death in the Western world, where the lifetime risk of dying from this disease is 1 : 50 (see Chapter 37).

Bacterial and amoebic **dysentery** affect the colon and are particularly common in travellers to endemic areas.

Ulcerative colitis only affects the colon and rectum, while Crohn's disease can also cause ileitis and peri-anal inflammation (see Chapter 34).

Colonic diverticulae may become impacted with faeces, and inflamed, causing pain; this is a condition known as **diverticulitis**. Blood vessels in diverticulae may be eroded, causing torrential haemorrhage. The pain of diverticulitis is usually felt in the **left lower quadrant** of the abdomen.

Polyps, cancer and vascular abnormalities (**angiodysplasia**) may cause anaemia.

Constipation, diarrhoea and abdominal pain are frequently due to the **irritable bowel syndrome** (IBS), without any evident organic pathology (see Chapter 29).

14 Rectum and anus

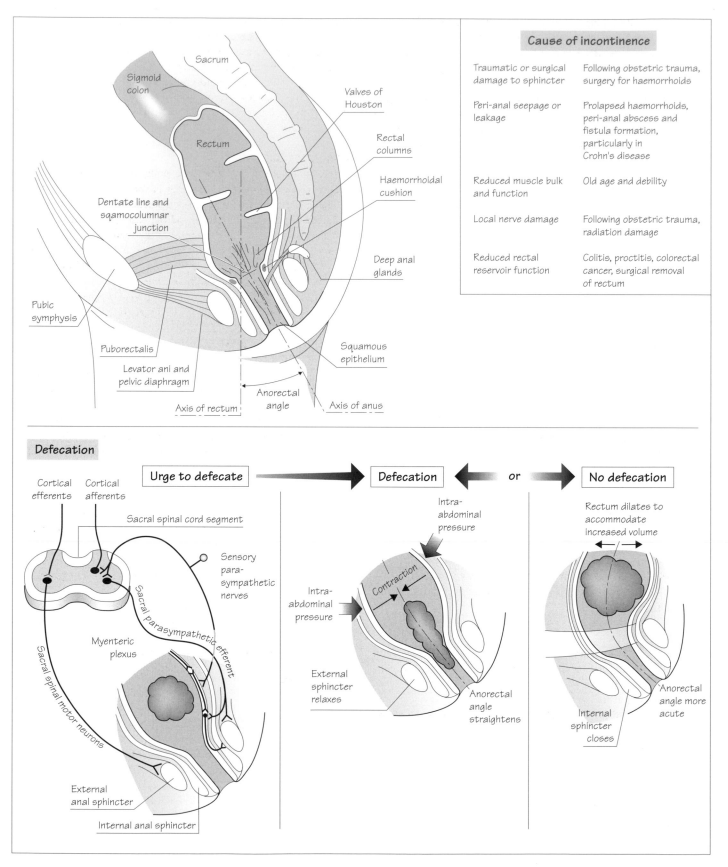

Cause of incontinence

Traumatic or surgical damage to sphincter	Following obstetric trauma, surgery for haemorrhoids
Peri-anal seepage or leakage	Prolapsed haemorrhoids, peri-anal abscess and fistula formation, particularly in Crohn's disease
Reduced muscle bulk and function	Old age and debility
Local nerve damage	Following obstetric trauma, radiation damage
Reduced rectal reservoir function	Colitis, proctitis, colorectal cancer, surgical removal of rectum

Labels (upper figure):
Sacrum, Sigmoid colon, Valves of Houston, Rectum, Rectal columns, Haemorrhoidal cushion, Dentate line and sqamocolumnar junction, Deep anal glands, Pubic symphysis, Squamous epithelium, Puborectalis, Levator ani and pelvic diaphragm, Anorectal angle, Axis of rectum, Axis of anus

Defecation

Urge to defecate → Defecation ← or → No defecation

Labels: Cortical efferents, Cortical afferents, Sacral spinal cord segment, Sensory para-sympathetic nerves, Sacral parasympathetic efferent, Myenteric plexus, Sacral spinal motor neurons, External anal sphincter, Internal anal sphincter

Intra-abdominal pressure, Contraction, External sphincter relaxes, Anorectal angle straightens

Rectum dilates to accommodate increased volume, Anorectal angle more acute, Internal sphincter closes

The rectum and anus comprise the most distal part of the gastrointestinal tract.

Structure

The rectum is **12 cm** long and extends from the **sigmoid colon** to the anus. It lies in front of the sacrum and is retroperitoneal, except proximally and anteriorly. It lies behind the **prostate** gland and seminal vesicles in men and behind the **pouch of Douglas**, uterus and vagina in women.

The wall of the rectum is similar to the colon, except that the longitudinal muscle layer is continuous. The mucosa is thrown into three semilunar transverse folds, known as the **valves of Houston**, which separate flatus from faeces and prevents them entering the distal rectum spontaneously.

Distally, the mucosa forms longitudinal ridges, called **rectal columns**, and the intervening furrows terminate in small folds at the anorectal junction, termed **anal valves**. The line through the anal valves is also the **squamocolumnar junction** between the rectal and anal mucosae and is termed the **dentate line**.

Three cushions of loose connective tissue are arranged circumferentially above the dentate line. They contain a venous plexus (**haemorrhoidal plexus**) and contribute to anal sphincter function. The veins enlarge with time, forming piles or haemorrhoids.

The anus is **2.5–4.0 cm** long and its lumen is directed posteriorly, forming a 70° angle with the rectal lumen. This **angulation** assists anal sphincter function. The circular smooth muscle layer, which is continuous with the rectal muscular layer, forms the powerful **internal anal sphincter**. An external layer of voluntary (striated) muscle constitutes the **external anal sphincter**. Muscle fibres of the **levator ani** and **puborectalis** muscles, which form part of the pelvic floor, encircle the anus; the levator ani lift the anus while the puborectalis pulls it forward and upward, making the **anorectal angle** more acute, further strengthening the sphincter.

The anus is lined by a **non-cornified stratified squamous epithelium** that is continuous with the peri-anal skin. **Submucosal anal glands** situated deep to the sphincter communicate with the surface through narrow ducts and their secretions lubricate and protect the anal canal.

Autonomic and **somatic nerves** from the sacral segments of the spinal cord innervate the rectum and anus. Internal anal sphincter tone is maintained by **parasympathetic** signals and the external anal sphincter is controlled by **sacral motor neurons**. The anus is innervated by somatic sensory nerve endings and is, therefore, as sensitive as the skin to pain and touch.

Function

The rectum acts as a **reservoir** for faeces and the anus is a powerful **sphincter** controlling defecation. The rectum is wider than the rest of the large intestine and can be further distended.

Defecation is initiated by distension of the rectum, causing increased **pressure**, which stimulates **intrinsic nerves** to increase **peristalsis** proximally in the sigmoid colon and to relax the **internal anal sphincter**. **Parasympathetic nerves** from the sacral plexus amplify this intrinsic neural reflex. The **external anal sphincter** is under voluntary control and if it relaxes when the internal anal sphincter relaxes, defecation commences. **Puborectalis** and **levator ani** relax, allowing the **anorectal angle** to straighten, and abdominal muscles contract, to increase **intra-abdominal pressure** and help expel faeces. Conversely, if the external anal sphincter does not relax, the urge to defecate passes.

Although the rectum does not normally absorb nutrients, medications can be administered by a **suppository** or an **enema** and are absorbed into the systemic circulation. This is particularly useful in babies and patients who cannot swallow.

Common disorders

Anorectal disorders typically cause **pain**, itching (**pruritis ani**) and bleeding (**haematochesia**). Pain can inhibit defecation, resulting in hardening of the stool and a self-perpetuating cycle of **constipation**. Inflammation causes **diarrhoea** and the passage of **mucus**. Chronic inflammation can reduce the ability of the rectum to dilate, causing **urgency** of defecation. **Tenesmus** is the sense of incomplete defecation. **Incontinence** is a distressing symptom, which may result from local disease, severe diarrhoea or neuromuscular disorders.

Bright red rectal bleeding occurring at the end of defecation is usually caused by haemorrhoids. Blood mixed with stool indicates bleeding from a more proximal source.

The anus can be examined externally to reveal prolapsed haemorrhoids, skin tags and anal fissure. To complete clinical examination of the anorectum, a gloved finger is inserted into the anus (**digital rectal examination**) and this can be followed by a **proctoscopy** or a **sigmoidoscopy** (see Chapters 43 & 44).

Cancer and **inflammation** affect the rectum as frequently as the remainder of the large intestine. In ulcerative colitis, **proctitis** (inflammation of the rectum) is almost invariably present. **Crohn's** disease does not always affect the rectum; however, anorectal Crohn's disease causing abscesses and fistulae occurs in 30% of cases (see Chapters 34 & 37).

Haemorrhoids are caused by engorgement of veins in the soft connective tissue cushions around the anorectal junction. First degree haemorrhoids remain within the rectum, second degree haemorrhoids reversibly prolapse out of the anus, and third degree haemorrhoids are permanently prolapsed.

Passage of hard stool against a tight anal sphincter can tear the anal skin, causing an **anal fissure**.

Abscesses and **fistulae** in the soft tissue around the anus are caused by infection of the peri-anal glands. They are treated with antibiotics and surgical incision and drainage.

Sexually transmitted diseases, including peri-anal warts caused by the human papilloma virus, genital herpes and syphilis may affect the anorectum.

Pain in the anus, without any discernable organic cause is **proctalgia fugax** (see Chapter 29).

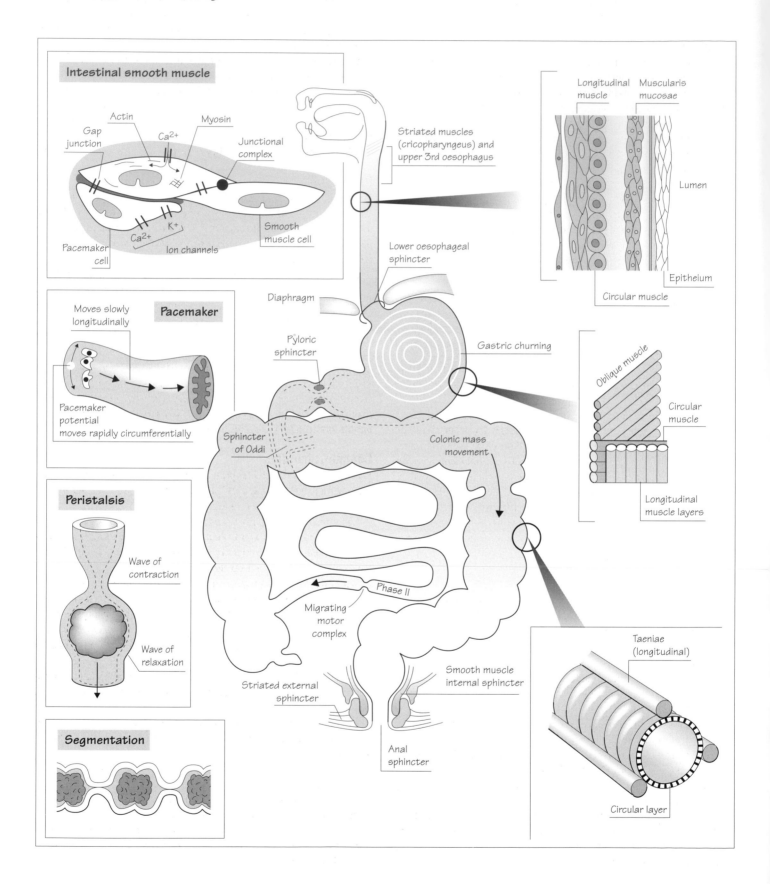

Intestinal smooth muscle

Gap junction

Actin

Myosin

Ca^{2+}

Junctional complex

Smooth muscle cell

Pacemaker cell

Ca^{2+}

K^+

Ion channels

Striated muscles (cricopharyngeus) and upper 3rd oesophagus

Longitudinal muscle

Muscularis mucosae

Lumen

Epitheium

Circular muscle

Lower oesophageal sphincter

Diaphragm

Pacemaker

Moves slowly longitudinally

Pacemaker potential moves rapidly circumferentially

Pyloric sphincter

Gastric churning

Oblique muscle

Circular muscle

Longitudinal muscle layers

Sphincter of Oddi

Colonic mass movement

Peristalsis

Wave of contraction

Wave of relaxation

Phase II

Migrating motor complex

Taeniae (longitudinal)

Striated external sphincter

Smooth muscle internal sphincter

Segmentation

Anal sphincter

Circular layer

Smooth muscle in the intestinal tract powers the disruption, mixing and propulsion of food from mouth to anus. It also discharges glandular contents and allows sphincters to separate intestinal compartments.

Structure

Apart from the mouth, tongue, pharynx and external anal sphincter, which have striated muscle under voluntary control, the gastrointestinal system contains **non-striated smooth muscle** under enteric and autonomic nervous control. Unusually, the upper oesophagus has striated muscle that is not under voluntary control.

The main muscle bulk is arranged in an **outer longitudinal layer** and an **inner circular layer**, allowing shortening and constriction of the hollow tube. In the caecum and colon, the longitudinal layer is bundled in **three separate cords** or **taenia**. An inner **oblique layer** augments these layers in the stomach and the circular layer is thickened around **sphincters**, increasing the constrictive force. The main sphincters are the lower oesophageal sphincter, the pylorus, the sphincter of Oddi, the ileocaecal valve and the anal sphincter.

A thin layer of muscle, the **muscularis mucosae**, separates the lamina propria from the submucosa.

Smooth muscle cells are **spindle-shaped** and lack striations created by organized bundles of actin and myosin.

Function

Contraction is mediated by **cross-linking of actin and myosin**, as in striated muscle. Contraction is initiated by increased intracellular Ca^{2+} concentration, which is regulated by hormonal and neural signals.

Intrinsic electric **pacemaker** cells are interspersed among the muscle cells and these provide a characteristic, **low frequency** wave of electrical depolarization and repolarization, known as the slow wave, that travels down the intestine. Pacemaker cells communicate via **gap junctions**, with the signal travelling faster circumferentially than transversely, so that a **synchronous** wave is propagated along the intestine. Distinct pacemaker frequencies characterize each organ; for example, the **gastric slow wave** frequency is three contractions per minute, which can be measured through electrodes on the abdominal wall (**electrogastrography**).

Tonic contractions

These are mainly **sustained**, low-pressure contractions that occur in organs with a major **storage** function, such as the gallbladder and rectum. High-pressure tonic activity characterizes **sphincters**.

Phasic contractions

These short-lived, rhythmic contractions predominate in the intestine. They are controlled by intrinsic pacemakers, autonomic nerves and coordinated reflex enteric nerve activity, and include:
• **Peristalsis**: which is a complex movement whereby a wave of muscular relaxation, followed by a wave of contraction, passes down the intestinal tract proximally to distally. The wave forces intestinal contents before it and is most prominent in the oesophagus, stomach and small intestine. In vomiting, peristaltic contractions move retrogradely (distally to proximally).
• **Gastric churning**: which is the result of tonic contraction of the pylorus and vigorous peristalsis in the stomach, repeatedly **squeezing and mixing** solid food, turning it into a **semi-liquid chyme** that is released into the duodenum.

• **Segmenting movements**: which are randomly spaced, **non-propagating** circular muscle contractions that mix intestinal contents.
• **Colonic mass movement**: which is a powerful, sweeping contraction that occurs a few times a day, forcing faeces into the rectum and stimulating defecation.
• **Interdigestive migrating motor complex** (**IMMC**): which comprises **three stages** lasting about an hour each, occurring between meals. In stage I, movement is absent. Stage II, comprising of random segmenting movements, is followed by stage III, which comprises a forceful wave of contraction that migrates from lower oesophagus to terminal ileum. This wave, sweeping the stomach and intestine clean of food debris, is termed the '**intestinal housekeeper**'.

Regulation

Peristalsis is intrinsic to the intestine, occurring even in surgically isolated segments, and is mediated by reflex enteric nerve activity. **Nitric oxide** (NO) is the main mediator of relaxation in the advancing front of a peristaltic wave, while **acetylcholine** (ACh) and other neurotransmitters mediate contraction.

Entero-endocrine and neural pathways mediate **reflex motility** involving spatially separated parts of the gastrointestinal system, such as the cholecystokinin-induced contraction of the gallbladder in response to food in the duodenum, the **gastrocolic** reflex (urge to defecate after eating) and the **ileal brake** (reduced ileal peristalsis when food reaches the distal small intestine).

Serotonin (5-hydroxytryptamine, **5HT**), released by entero-endocrine cells, is a critical regulator of intestinal motility through its effects on enteric neurons. $5HT_3$ receptors mediate increased intestinal motility, while $5HT_4$ receptors mediate the opposite effect, and selective inhibitors could prove to be useful therapeutically.

Common disorders

Dysmotility may manifest as **pain**, **discomfort**, **early satiety**, **vomiting**, **diarrhoea** or **constipation**. It is associated with some rare but serious conditions and some more common conditions.

Oesophageal dysmotility can cause pain (odynophagia) and difficulty in swallowing (**dysphagia**). Powerful, uncoordinated spasms (**nutcracker oesophagus**) can cause severe pain. In **achalasia**, tonic hyperactivity of the lower oesophageal sphincter, and absent peristalsis proximally, causes dysphagia and dilatation of the distal oesophagus.

Infants may develop gastric outlet obstruction with persistent projectile vomiting due to congenital **hypertrophy** of the **pyloric sphincter**.

Following surgery or severe illness, generalized paralysis of the intestine, known as **paralytic ileus**, may develop. This is aggravated by hypokalaemia, hypocalcaemia and the use of opiates, which inhibit intestinal motility. It usually resolves spontaneously, although the intestine may dilate to such an extent that the wall becomes ischaemic and emergency surgery is necessary.

Less well-defined abnormalities of motility may contribute to **slow-transit constipation**, functional bowel disorders and **irritable bowel syndrome** (IBS).

Muscular spasm may be treated medically with relaxants such as mebeverine and hyoscine. Sphincter spasm may be mechanically **dilated** or **botulinum toxin** injections may induce temporary paralysis. Both techniques are used to treat achalasia.

Metoclopramide may stimulate foregut motility, as may **erythromycin**, acting on motilin receptors, and **neostigmine**, acting on muscarinic acetylcholine receptors.

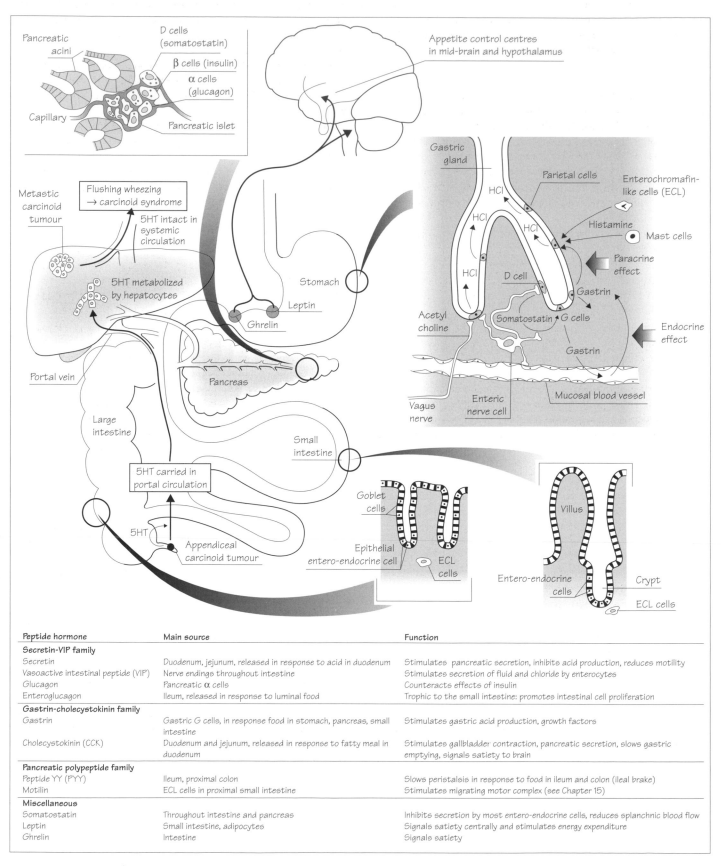

Peptide hormone	Main source	Function
Secretin-VIP family		
Secretin	Duodenum, jejunum, released in response to acid in duodenum	Stimulates pancreatic secretion, inhibits acid production, reduces motility
Vasoactive intestinal peptide (VIP)	Nerve endings throughout intestine	Stimulates secretion of fluid and chloride by enterocytes
Glucagon	Pancreatic α cells	Counteracts effects of insulin
Enteroglucagon	Ileum, released in response to luminal food	Trophic to the small intestine: promotes intestinal cell proliferation
Gastrin-cholecystokinin family		
Gastrin	Gastric G cells, in response food in stomach, pancreas, small intestine	Stimulates gastric acid production, growth factors
Cholecystokinin (CCK)	Duodenum and jejunum, released in response to fatty meal in duodenum	Stimulates gallbladder contraction, pancreatic secretion, slows gastric emptying, signals satiety to brain
Pancreatic polypeptide family		
Peptide YY (PYY)	Ileum, proximal colon	Slows peristalsis in response to food in ileum and colon (ileal brake)
Motilin	ECL cells in proximal small intestine	Stimulates migrating motor complex (see Chapter 15)
Miscellaneous		
Somatostatin	Throughout intestine and pancreas	Inhibits secretion by most entero-endocrine cells, reduces splanchnic blood flow
Leptin	Small intestine, adipocytes	Signals satiety centrally and stimulates energy expenditure
Ghrelin	Intestine	Signals satiety

The first hormone ever discovered was the enteric hormone **secretin**. Subsequently, over 30 enteric (or gut) hormones have been described, all secreted by specialized entero-endocrine (also called neuro-endocrine) cells distributed throughout the gastrointestinal system. They mainly control gastrointestinal motility and secretion, and they mediate communication from one part of the intestine to another and outside the intestine, for example, to the central nervous system.

Structure
Entero-endocrine cells
The entero-endocrine system is **diffusely** distributed. Most entero-endocrine cells are found in the **epithelium** of the intestine. They vary in shape, although most are pyramidal with the base of the pyramid on the basement membrane, where prominent **secretory granules** are located. Some cells span the epithelium, with the apex in contact with the lumen, while others do not. **Entero-chromaffin-like cells** (ECL) are similar in structure but are located in the submucosa or in the pancreatic islets.

Many entero-endocrine cells contain more than one hormone, and hormones are preferentially distributed in cells in different parts of the system. Enteric hormones are also found in **neurons** in the enteric and central nervous systems and are, therefore, often called **gut-brain peptides**. Endocrine and neuro-endocrine effects in the gastrointestinal system therefore often overlap.

Enteric hormones
Almost all entero-endocrine cells contain **serotonin** (5-hydroxytryptamine, **5HT**), in addition to peptide hormones, while ECL cells contain **histamine**. Most enteric hormones are **short peptides** that are synthesized as larger prepropeptides and modified by, for example, cleavage, amidation and sulphation. They fall into **structural families** and tissue distribution and function vary widely (see table in figure opposite).

Function
Enteric hormones perform a great range of functions and work in different ways. Some are relatively well understood and others are only now beginning to be understood. The functions of some peptide hormones are shown in the table opposite.

Enteric hormones may act locally (**paracrine** action) in the immediate vicinity of where they are secreted; for example, **somatostatin** produced by D cells in pancreatic islets inhibit insulin and glucagon secretion. They may also first enter the circulation and then be transported to targets in other parts of the intestine (**endocrine** action). An example is **cholecystokinin** (CCK) released by cells in the duodenum and then inhibiting gastric gastrin production and stimulating gallbladder contraction. They may also be transported to other organs and, in particular, to the **central nervous system**. **Leptin** and **ghrelin** are recently discovered examples, which signal satiety, and are involved in the control of nutrition.

Individual hormones may also have different effects on different targets, sometimes mediated by separate **receptors**. Examples include gastrin, which binds to CCK-A and CCK-B receptors, and 5HT, which has at least five different receptors ($5HT_{1-5}$ receptors), sometimes mediating opposite effects.

Some enteric hormones and their receptors have very specific effects that have been successfully targeted therapeutically. **Histamine receptor type 2** (H2R) antagonists, such as cimetidine and ranitidine, that reduce gastric acid secretion, are among the most successful agents of this type.

Similarly, **octreotide**, a modified octapeptide (8 amino acid) homologue of **somatostatin**, is widely used to inhibit the secretion of other enteric hormones, inhibit intestinal exocrine secretion and reduce splanchnic blood flow.

There are now also new agents aimed at inhibiting different 5HT receptors, to treat aspects of the irritable bowel syndrome (IBS).

Attempts to use **leptin** to decrease appetite and induce **weight loss** have been generally unsuccessful; however, now that the role of enteric hormones in regulating body mass has been appreciated, this is a challenging and promising area of clinical research.

Common disorders
Subtle entero-endocrine dysfunction may be responsible for very common conditions such as the irritable bowel syndrome and obesity; however, this is hard to prove and remains speculative.

Most serious entero-endocrine diseases are **rare**, although clinically silent carcinoid tumours are frequently noted at autopsy.

Symptoms caused by disorders of the entero-endocrine system are protean, reflecting the many effects of enteric hormones. To diagnose entero-endocrine dysfunction, **circulating enteric hormone levels** may be measured (in the fasting state, as feeding alters the levels of most hormones) and excess 5HT secretion may be determined by measuring urinary excretion of 5-hydroxyindole acetic acid (**5-HIAA**).

Carcinoid tumours arise from entero-endocrine cells, and are relatively common. They may secrete a variety of hormones and growth factors and 5HT secretion is usually prominent. Carcinoids usually arise in the appendix, but may occur in other parts of the intestine. The portal circulation delivers 5HT from intestinal carcinoids to the liver, which efficiently clears it, so that patients remain asymptomatic. However, when the tumours metastasize to the liver and deliver their hormones directly into the systemic circulation, they give rise to the **carcinoid syndrome**, characterized by episodes of **flushing** caused by release of 5HT and **fibrosis** of the heart and peripheral tissues, caused by growth factors, such as transforming growth factor β (**TGFβ**) released by the tumour.

G-cell tumours (**gastrinomas**) secrete excess gastrin, causing the **Zollinger–Ellison syndrome**, which is characterized by severe gastric hyperacidity, recurrent peptic ulceration and malabsorption due to the reduced efficiency of digestive enzymes in an acid milieu. Gastrinomas may occur sporadically, or in association with other endocrine tumours in a syndrome known as **multiple endocrine neoplasia I**, or MEN-I. The syndrome is caused by an inherited abnormality in the tumour suppressor gene *MEN1*.

There are many other rare entero-endocrine tumour syndromes, such as **glucagonomas** and vasoactive intestinal peptide (**VIP**)-secreting tumours that cause the syndrome of watery diarrhoea and hypokalaemia (**Werner–Morrison syndrome**) (see Chapter 38).

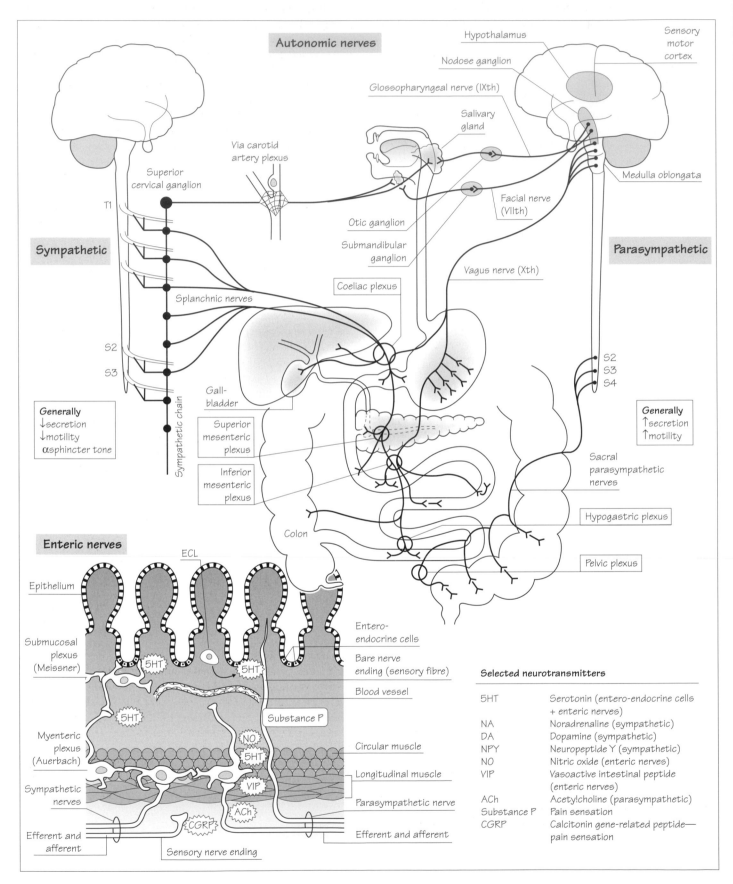

Autonomic nerves

Sympathetic

Generally
↓secretion
↓motility
αsphincter tone

Parasympathetic

Generally
↑secretion
↑motility

Hypothalamus

Sensory motor cortex

Nodose ganglion

Glossopharyngeal nerve (IXth)

Salivary gland

Medulla oblongata

Via carotid artery plexus

Superior cervical ganglion

T1

Otic ganglion

Submandibular ganglion

Facial nerve (VIIth)

Vagus nerve (Xth)

Coeliac plexus

Splanchnic nerves

S2

S3

Sympathetic chain

Gall-bladder

Superior mesenteric plexus

Inferior mesenteric plexus

Colon

S2
S3
S4

Sacral parasympathetic nerves

Hypogastric plexus

Pelvic plexus

Enteric nerves

ECL

Epithelium

Submucosal plexus (Meissner)

5HT

5HT

5HT

Entero-endocrine cells

Bare nerve ending (sensory fibre)

Blood vessel

Substance P

Myenteric plexus (Auerbach)

NO
5HT
VIP
ACh
CGRP

Circular muscle

Longitudinal muscle

Sympathetic nerves

Parasympathetic nerve

Efferent and afferent

Efferent and afferent

Sensory nerve ending

Selected neurotransmitters

5HT	Serotonin (entero-endocrine cells + enteric nerves)
NA	Noradrenaline (sympathetic)
DA	Dopamine (sympathetic)
NPY	Neuropeptide Y (sympathetic)
NO	Nitric oxide (enteric nerves)
VIP	Vasoactive intestinal peptide (enteric nerves)
ACh	Acetylcholine (parasympathetic)
Substance P	Pain sensation
CGRP	Calcitonin gene-related peptide—pain sensation

Neural as well as hormonal signals coordinate gastrointestinal function, including motility, and the gastrointestinal system has its own intrinsic enteric nervous system, as well as being innervated by the sympathetic and parasympathetic divisions of the autonomic nervous system.

Structure

Enteric nervous system

There are between 10^7 and 10^8 nerve cells in the enteric nervous system, which almost matches the number in the spinal cord. Most are small, with **short processes** that terminate locally, and they are generally arranged in two layers: the **myenteric** (Auerbach's) plexus that lies between the circular and longitudinal muscle layers and the **submucosal** (Meissner's) plexus that lies in the submucosa. The submucosal plexus mainly responds to and regulates **epithelial cell** and submucosal **blood vessel** function, while the myenteric plexus mainly regulates intestinal **motility** and **sphincter** function.

Enteric nerves typically use more than one **neurotransmitter**, including a variety of amino acid derivatives, **peptides**, **acetylcholine (ACh)**, and **nitric oxide** (NO). There may also be **multiple receptor types** for any one neurotransmitter; for example, there are at least five different subtypes of serotonin (5-hydroxytryptamine, **5HT**) receptors. Enteric nerves respond to stimuli from other enteric nerves, from autonomic nerves, and from epithelial cells, including entero-endocrine cells.

Extrinsic motor (efferent) nerves

Voluntary nerves

Voluntary nerves control the lips, tongue, muscles of mastication, as well as pelvic floor muscles and the external anal sphincter.

Autonomic nerves

Sympathetic nerves originating from the **cervical sympathetic chain** and travelling in the **splanchnic nerves**, via the coeliac and other **ganglia**, innervate the entire gastrointestinal system.

Parasympathetic innervation is provided mainly via the **glossopharyngeal** (IXth) and **vagus** (Xth) cranial nerves to foregut and mid-gut structures. The salivary glands also receive parasympathetic fibres via the **facial** (VIIth) cranial nerve. The **sacral parasympathetic plexus** provides parasympathetic innervation distally beyond the hepatic flexure of the colon.

Extrinsic sensory (afferent) nerves

Touch, **pain and temperature** sensation in the mouth and tongue are similar to those in the skin and are represented on the **sensory cortex** in the same way. In fact the tongue has a relatively large cortical representation. Similarly, somatic sensory nerves innervate the **anus**. **Taste** sensation is carried by fibres that synapse in the nucleus of the **tractus solitarius** in the mid-brain.

Sensory information from the rest of the gastrointestinal system travels to the central nervous system via the **sympathetic** and **parasympathetic** nerves. Most enteric vagal fibres are afferent; nonetheless, the density of sensory nerves in the internal organs is much lower than, for example, the skin. Visceral afferents send signals to the **hypothalamus**, where some **pain** sensation is processed and also to centres controlling **swallowing**, **vomiting**, **blood pressure**, **heart rate** and other autonomic functions. Afferent nerves use **substance P** and calcitonin gene-related peptide (**CGRP**) as transmitters.

Function

Complex motor functions, such as **peristalsis**, remain intact in isolated intestinal segments lacking external innervation, confirming the complexity and completeness of the enteric nervous system. Enteric nerves also control other important functions, including **secretion** and regulation of **blood flow** under the changing conditions imposed by intermittent feeding. Their function is, however, modified by autonomic innervation. Sympathetic nerves, using **noradrenaline (NA)**, **dopamine (DA)** and **neuropeptide Y (PY)** as transmitters, tend to decrease intestinal motility and secretion and increase sphincter tone. Parasympathetic nerves mainly use **acetylcholine (ACh)** and **cholecystokinin (CCK)** as neurotransmitters and tend to increase secretion and motility.

Although there is some spatial coding of visceral sensory input in the central nervous system, **visceral sensation** is spatially and temporally much **less precise** than somatic sensation. Many factors contribute to this, including the relative **low density** of sensory nerves in the intestine and other internal organs, and the fact that visceral afferent nerves use non-specific **naked nerve endings** rather than specialized sensory organs, such as the touch, temperature and pain receptors found in the skin, so that they cannot differentiate widely divergent stimuli. Furthermore, visceral afferent fibres are **unmyelinated** and relatively slow-conducting, so temporal resolution is reduced.

The poor resolution and specificity of visceral sensation contributes to difficulty in localizing visceral pain and is partly responsible for the phenomenon of **referred pain**. This is illustrated by the classic symptom pattern in evolving **acute appendicitis**. The earliest symptoms include **peri-umbilical abdominal pain**, anorexia and **nausea**, which are mediated by visceral nerves serving the entire mid-gut. As inflammation progresses and the visceral and parietal **peritoneum** are involved, somatic nerves innervating the parietal peritoneum are stimulated and pain is localized to the **right iliac fossa**, overlying the inflamed organ. Finally, muscles overlying the region become tense, causing **guarding**, a protective reflex mediated by motor nerves to voluntary muscle (see Chapter 12).

Common disorders

Abnormalities of enteric and autonomic nerve function can contribute to many typical gastrointestinal symptoms, including **nausea**, **vomiting**, **diarrhoea**, **constipation** and abdominal **pain**. Dysfunction of the enteric nervous system, causing increased visceral sensitivity and abnormal motility and secretion, may contribute to **functional bowel disorders** and the irritable bowel syndrome (IBS), although there is no definitive proof of this.

Diabetes mellitus and other systemic illnesses can damage peripheral nerves in the intestine causing **autonomic neuropathy**.

Hirschsprung's syndrome is a rare disorder caused by the congenital absence of **myenteric nerves** in a segment of the colon, causing chronic, severe constipation. Patients may develop a massively dilated, faeces-filled colon (**megacolon**) proximal to the affected segment and surgical removal of the affected segment is curative.

Visceral pain may sometimes be treated by ablation of the sympathetic autonomic nerves to the affected part; for example, in chronic pancreatitis, the coeliac ganglion may be removed or destroyed *in situ*.

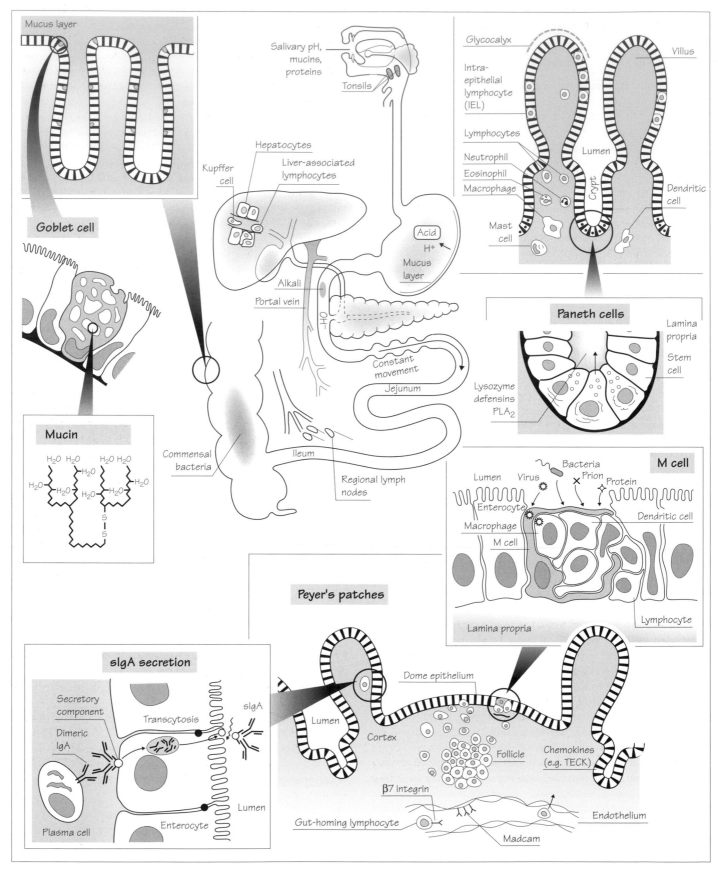

Mucus layer

Goblet cell

Mucin

H_2O H_2O H_2O H_2O
H_2O H_2O H_2O H_2O
H_2O H_2O H_2O

S
S

Salivary pH, mucins, proteins

Tonsils

Hepatocytes

Liver-associated lymphocytes

Kupffer cell

Alkali

Portal vein

HCO₃

Acid
H⁺
Mucus layer

Constant movement

Jejunum

Commensal bacteria

Ileum

Regional lymph nodes

Glycocalyx

Intra-epithelial lymphocyte (IEL)

Lymphocytes

Neutrophil
Eosinophil
Macrophage

Mast cell

Villus

Lumen

Crypt

Dendritic cell

Paneth cells

Lamina propria

Stem cell

Lysozyme defensins PLA_2

M cell

Lumen Virus Bacteria Prion Protein

Enterocyte

Macrophage

M cell

Dendritic cell

Lymphocyte

Lamina propria

Peyer's patches

sIgA secretion

Secretory component

Transcytosis

sIgA

Dimeric IgA

Plasma cell

Enterocyte

Lumen

Dome epithelium

Lumen

Cortex

Follicle

Chemokines (e.g. TECK)

β7 integrin

Gut-homing lymphocyte

Madcam

Endothelium

The gastrointestinal system presents a large exposed surface area that must be maintained and defended. Furthermore, prions, viruses, bacteria, parasites, inert particles and toxins are constantly ingested and there is a large resident microbial flora, particularly in the large intestine. The mucosal immune system regulates how the body responds to these challenges.

Structure

Many structures contribute to gastrointestinal defences. Innate defence mechanisms include:

- The constant **movement** of intestinal contents, and their periodic expulsion.
- The **pH** and chemical composition of intestinal secretions; for example, corrosive stomach acid and detergent **bile salts**.
- Antibacterial enzymes and peptides, such as **lysozyme** in saliva and other exocrine secretions.
- **Mucins** form a tough, slippery mucous gel, protecting epithelial cells from mechanical damage.
- Intrinsic **cellular defences** in epithelial cells, which can resist and limit invasion by pathogens.
- Specialized intestinal epithelial cells, such as **Paneth cells**, which secrete many antibacterial enzymes and peptides, such as **defensins**.
- **Mast cells**, **eosinophils**, **neutrophils**, **macrophages** and **dendritic cells** in the lamina propria constitute a first line of defence against pathogens that breach the epithelial layer and also process and **present antigens** to cells of the adaptive immune system.

Adaptive immunedefences include:

- **Lamina propria lymphocytes**: these B and T cells are distinct from those found in the blood and are specifically targeted to the intestine.
- **Intra-epithelial lymphocytes**: T lymphocytes are found between epithelial cells, particularly in the small intestine. They are not migrating through, but are resident in this position. Many of these cells express γδ **T-cell receptors**, with a restricted repertoire, rather than the regular αβ T-cell receptors found elsewhere. They react to **lipid antigens** presented on CD1 cell surface molecules rather than peptides presented on classic major histocompatibility complex (MHC) class I or II molecules, and may have a special role responding to proteolipid antigens in bacterial cell membranes.
- **Peyer's patches**: these are distinctive structures with a specialized epithelial lining, containing B and T lymphocytes and antigen presenting cells. They are most numerous in the terminal ileum. The specialized **dome epithelium** lacks villi and crypts and the glycocalyx formed by microvilli and membrane glycoproteins is deficient. It contains specialized epithelial cells called **microfold** or **M cells**, which lack microvilli and contain membranous folds enclosing lymphocytes, macrophages and dendritic cells. They trap antigens and transport them across the epithelium, to interact with immune cells.

Under the dome epithelium, lymphocytes, macrophages and dendritic cells form a loose T-cell-rich **cortical region** and compact B-cell-rich **follicles**, resembling the organization of lymph nodes.

- **Tonsils** are lymphoid aggregates surrounding the opening of the hypopharynx, with a broadly similar structure and function to Peyer's patches, and in the stomach, colon and **appendix**, Peyer's patches may be substituted by less well-defined lymphoid aggregates in the lamina propria.

Function

While host defences must prevent infection and damage to the absorptive epithelium of the gastrointestinal tract, the **commensal** flora of the intestine is essential for health and the system must distinguish between beneficial and harmful bacteria. Furthermore, while the intestine must mount immune responses to pathogens, it must also prevent reactivity to food antigens to avoid **allergies** and **hypersensitivity**. The mucosal immune system fulfils these functions in ways that are still poorly understood. Thus while pathogens are generally repelled, **oral tolerance** develops towards to harmless intestinal contents.

- **M cells**. These transport intact peptides, viruses and bacteria across the epithelium and pass them on to antigen processing and presenting cells. The surface molecules involved in this transport are presently unknown.
- **Mucosal homing**. Antigens taken orally are transported to regional lymph nodes where they cause proliferation of lymphocytes. These specific T lymphocytes and antibody-producing B lymphocytes leave the lymph nodes and return to mucosal surfaces.

Homing to the mucosa is mediated by cell surface molecules that interact with receptors on blood vessels in the gastrointestinal tract (**addressins**). Lymphocytes homing to the intestine express the α4β7 **integrin** molecule that interacts with the mucosal addressin-cell adhesion molecule (**MAD-CAM**). Specific cytokines (chemokines) also attract subsets of lymphocytes to different parts of the intestine; for example, thymus and epithelial expressed chemokine (**TECK**) attracts cells to the small intestine.

- **Secretory dimeric immunoglobulin A (sIgA)**. Most B cells at mucosal surfaces produce IgA, which is the most abundant immunoglobulin in bronchial, reproductive tract and intestinal secretions. Two IgA molecules, joined together to form polymeric IgA (**pIgA**), bind to a receptor called **secretory component** (SC) on the basolateral surfaces of epithelia. The complex is transported across the cell cytoplasm (**transcytosed**) and sIgA is released at the luminal surface, by proteolytic cleavage of SC.

Common disorders

The intestinal epithelium is not impervious to proteins, viruses and bacteria, as was previously assumed. Prions, such as the bovine spongiform encephalopathy (**BSE**) **agent**, viruses, such as human immunodeficiency virus (**HIV**), and pathogenic bacteria, such as *Shigella*, are taken up by M cells, allowing systemic spread and **infection**.

Selective **IgA deficiency** affects about 1 : 500 people, without much effect on enteric immunity.

Chronic immune stimulation, for example, by *Helicobacter pylori* or by coeliac disease, can lead to excess proliferation of immune cells, neoplastic change and intestinal **lymphoma**.

True **food allergies** are rare, although they may be becoming more frequent; particularly those caused by nut antigens.

Dysregulated immune responses are implicated in **coeliac disease**, where there is hypersensitivity to peptides derived from wheat and other cereals and in **inflammatory bowel disease (IBD)**. Inflammation may normally be actively prevented by subsets of T lymphocytes, which might have regulatory functions that are defective in IBD.

19 Digestion and absorption

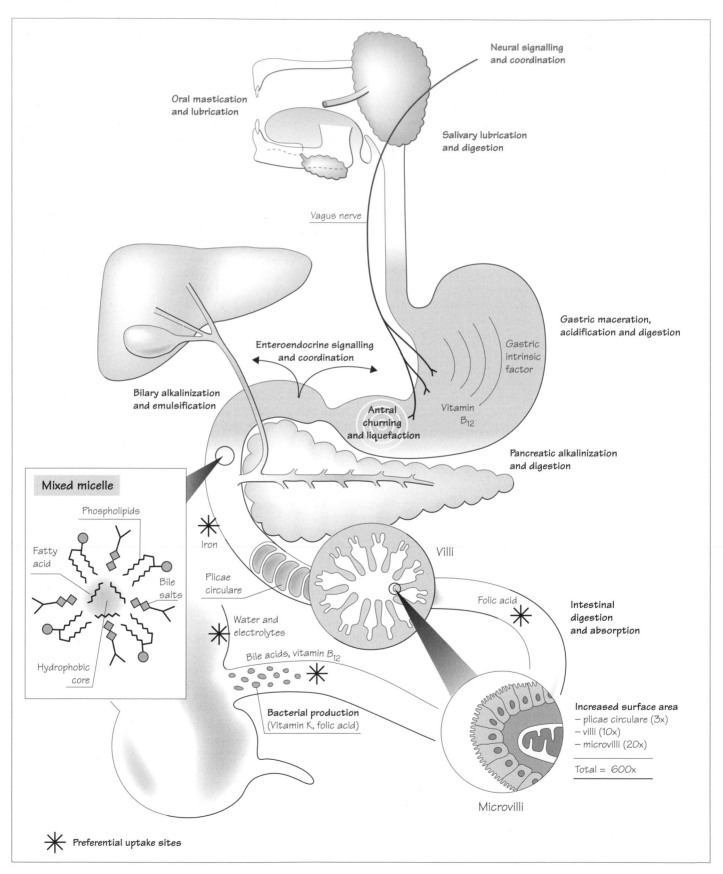

Neural signalling and coordination

Oral mastication and lubrication

Salivary lubrication and digestion

Vagus nerve

Gastric maceration, acidification and digestion

Gastric intrinsic factor

Vitamin B$_{12}$

Enteroendocrine signalling and coordination

Bilary alkalinization and emulsification

Antral churning and liquefaction

Pancreatic alkalinization and digestion

Mixed micelle

Phospholipids

Fatty acid

Bile salts

Hydrophobic core

Iron

Plicae circulare

Water and electrolytes

Bile acids, vitamin B$_{12}$

Villi

Folic acid

Intestinal digestion and absorption

Increased surface area
– plicae circulare (3x)
– villi (10x)
– microvilli (20x)

Total = 600x

Microvilli

Bacterial production
(Vitamin K, folic acid)

✳ Preferential uptake sites

The main function of the intestine is to digest and absorb nutrients, and it is variously adapted for this. Taste provides a guide to the nutritional value or potential toxicity of food, and while the colon is not essential for nutrition it helps to conserve water and salts. Details of digestion and absorption are considered in Chapters 20 and 21 and here general principles are emphasized.

Coordination

Hunting, gathering and supermarket shopping all require exquisite **neuromuscular coordination**, as do **biting**, **chewing** and **swallowing**. Thus, patients who are weak or who have neurological disease, such as a stroke, can rapidly become malnourished. Once food passes from the mouth to the oesophagus, the involuntary **enteric** and autonomic **nervous** systems and **hormones** produced by the **entero-endocrine** system coordinate digestion and absorption.

Motility

Food moves progressively through the intestine aided by **peristalsis**, which is modified by neuronal and endocrine signals. Antegrade movement is complemented by **churning** in the stomach, which mixes and pulverizes food into **chyme**, and the action of **sphincters**, which separate food into appropriate compartments. For example, the pyloric sphincter keeps food in the stomach until it is the correct consistency for digestion in the duodenum.

Mechanical disruption

Many foods are hard and irregular and could damage the delicate intestinal lining. The tough **oral epithelium** and **teeth** break and grind food into small pieces, while **saliva** moistens and lubricates it. Particle sizes are further reduced in the **stomach**, where powerful muscular **churning** converts food into a thick suspension called **chyme**. Reducing the size of food particles increases the **surface area to volume ratio**, enhancing the action of digestive enzymes. Chyme remains liquid until it reaches the large intestine, where waste is converted into semi-solid faeces by water reabsorption.

Solubilization

Food must be dissolved in an aqueous medium for digestive enzymes to act and while some fluid is ingested, most of the liquid in the intestinal lumen is actively **secreted** by the intestine and exocrine glands. It is subsequently **reabsorbed**, to maintain fluid balance.

Emulsification and micelle formation

Most dietary fat is too hydrophobic to dissolve in water, so mixing in the **alkaline** intestinal lumen emulsifies it, creating tiny particles and increasing the surface area available for lipid-digesting enzymes. **Amphiphilic bile salts**, phospholipids and cholesterol esters secreted in **bile** form micelles, which are microscopic particles with a hydrophobic core and the hydrophilic parts of the molecules on the outside. Digested lipids, such as fatty acids, partition into the hydrophobic core and can be absorbed from the intestinal lumen.

Acidification and alkalization

Optimal digestion in the stomach requires an acid environment, created by **HCl**, secreted by gastric parietal cells. Conversely, optimal digestion by pancreatic enzymes requires an alkaline medium, provided by HCO_3^-, secreted in the **bile** and **pancreatic juice**.

Enzymes

Enzymes are the most critical element of digestion, enabling chemically complex, polymeric foods to be processed to absorbable **monomers** at physiological temperatures and in a reasonable timescale.

Enzymatic digestion starts in the mouth with **salivary amylase**, which breaks down starch to form sugars. Stomach acid inhibits amylase activity and activates gastric pepsinogen to form **pepsin**, thus initiating protein digestion. Most enzymatic digestion takes place in the duodenum and jejunum, where **pancreatic** and **small intestinal** enzymes act in an alkaline milieu. The pancreas produces a prodigious amount and variety of digestive enzymes, including **proteinases**, **amylases**, **lipases** and **nucleases**, and pancreatic failure invariably causes malabsorption and malnutrition.

Enzymes can potentially digest components of the cells that produce them (**autodigestion**); therefore, many are synthesized as inactive **pro-enzymes**. Other enzymes activate them by proteolytic cleavage; for example, pancreatic trypsinogen (pro-enzyme) is cleaved to trypsin by enterokinase secreted by duodenal enterocytes.

Enterocytes contribute a critical final stage of enzyme digestion, whereby **brush-border disaccharidases** and **peptidases** attached to their apical surfaces break down partially digested sugars and peptides to absorbable monomers and oligomers.

Within enterocytes, enzymes continue the digestive process; for example, fatty acids are **reconstituted** into **triglycerides** and assembled into **chylomicrons** before export at the basolateral membrane and transport to the circulation via lymphatic channels.

Special factors

Intrinsic factor is a glycoprotein produced by the stomach, which binds **vitamin B_{12}**, protecting it from breakdown in the proximal intestine. In the terminal ileum, vitamin B_{12} is released and absorbed. Similar systems operate for other essential minerals and vitamins. Some nutrients, for example, **vitamin K**, may be synthesized in the intestine by commensal **bacteria**.

Surface area

Absorption of digested food depends critically on a well-adapted and ample surface area. The **small intestine** is the main absorptive surface, although some substances can be absorbed through the **oral mucosa** and others in the **stomach** (e.g. alcohol, which notoriously 'goes straight to the head').

Plicae circulare are transverse folds, which increase the surface area threefold, and **villi** are finger-like projections into the lumen, which increase intestinal surface area 10-fold. **Microvilli**, which are microscopic, finger-like projections on the apical surface of enterocytes, increase the absorptive surface area 20-fold, so that overall the surface area is increased **600×** over that of a simple hollow tube.

Specialized absorptive surfaces

Enterocytes are exquisitely adapted for absorption by expressing the appropriate cell membrane **transporters** and **channels**. In addition, sections of the intestine are **specialized** for absorbing particular nutrients; for example, **folic acid** is mostly absorbed in the **jejunum** and **vitamin B_{12}** and **bile acids** are mostly absorbed in the **terminal ileum**.

Enterocytes can regulate the extent of absorption; for example, **iron** transport is inhibited when there are sufficient body stores and, in genetic **haemochromatosis**, regulation malfunctions and patients accumulate iron.

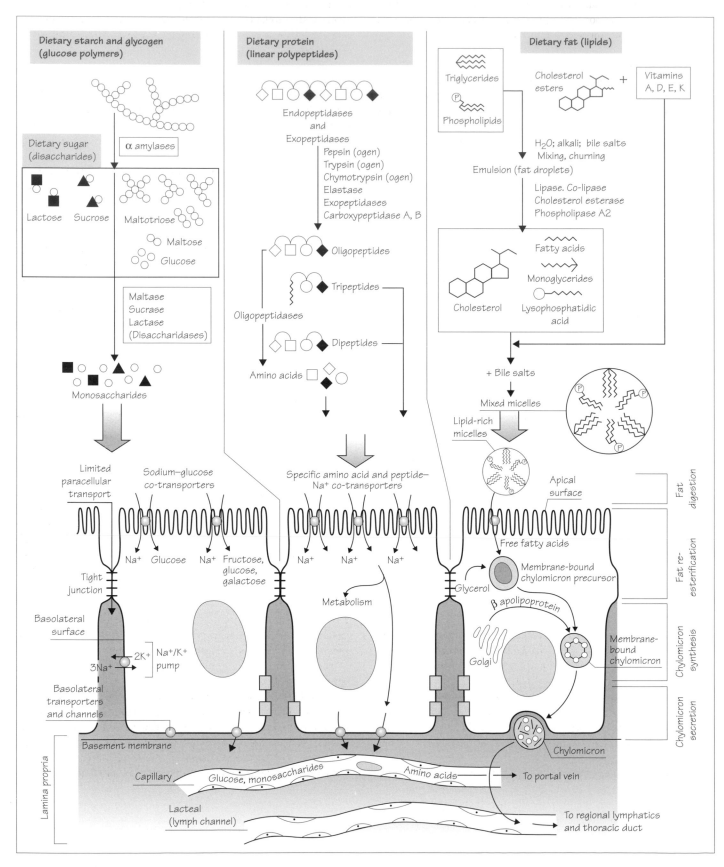

Carbohydrates, proteins and lipids form the major part of the diet and are known as **macronutrients**, in contrast to **micronutrients**, such as vitamins, which are only needed in milligram or microgram quantities. Macronutrients provide all the dietary energy and most of the structural materials needed for body tissues. Robust mechanisms efficiently extract and absorb macronutrients from the diet.

Carbohydrates

Carbohydrates are ingested as **starches** and **sugars**, which are longer or shorter polymers of monosaccharides. Plant starch is a complex, branched polysaccharide of glucose linked by $\alpha1$–4 and $\alpha1$–6 glycosidic linkages, while cane sugar (**sucrose**) is a disaccharide composed of **glucose** and **fructose**. **Lactose**, the major sugar in milk, is composed of glucose and **galactose**. Humans cannot digest $\beta1$–4 glycosidic linkages in cellulose, the major polysaccharide in plant cell walls, which is also known as dietary **fibre** or **roughage**.

Polysaccharides are digested by **amylases**. Although some amylase is produced by **salivary** glands, most digestion is performed by **pancreatic** amylase. Amylases produce monosaccharides (glucose), disaccharides (maltose) and maltotriose, and limit dextrins with short branches; however, enterocytes can only absorb monosaccharides. **Oligosaccharidases**, such as **sucrase**, **maltase** and **lactase**, produced by enterocytes are present in the **brush border** and perform the final digestion of dissaccharides and trisaccharides to monosaccharides.

Specific transporters, such as the **sodium–glucose co-transporter** (**SGLT-1**), in the apical surface of enterocytes, transport monosaccharides into the cytoplasm. The enterocyte cytoplasm is constantly depleted of sodium by the basolaterally situated Na^+/K^+ pump that pumps two K^+ ions into the cell in exchange for three Na^+ ions, using energy derived from the hydrolysis of adenosine triphosphate (ATP). This adenosine triphosphatase (ATPase) also maintains a small negative electric potential within the cell. The **electrogenic and osmotic Na^+ gradient** generated by the Na^+/K^+ ATPase is used to transport monosaccharides, amino acids and bile salts into the cytoplasm using different Na^+-coupled transporters. This co-transport of Na^+ ions and sugars is used clinically in the composition of **oral rehydration solution**, which combines glucose and salt, so that Na^+, which is depleted by, for example, gastroenteritis, is replaced when enterocytes absorb Na^+ together with glucose.

Absorbed monosaccharides leave the enterocyte by **facilitated diffusion**, through **selective channels** in the **basolateral** surface. They then enter the circulation via the rich **capillary network** in the villus.

Proteins

Protein digestion begins in the stomach with the action of **pepsin**, although the **pancreas** secretes the bulk of important **proteases**. **Trypsinogen**, **chymotrypsinogen** and **proelastase** are **endopeptidases** that cleave at specific residues in the peptide chain, while the **carboxypeptidases** A and B are **exopeptidases** that remove single amino acids from the carboxyl terminal, leaving short **oligopeptides**. **Enterokinase** is an enterocyte-derived endopeptidase that activates trypsinogen. Trypsin then can activate other molecules of trypsinogen (**autocatalysis**).

Enterocyte-derived **peptidases** in the **brush border** complete the digestion of peptides, producing single amino acids and di- and tripeptides that are absorbed. Amino acids enter enterocytes along with Na^+ ions, using **five** different **co-transporters** that are **selective** for neutral, aromatic, imino, positively charged and negatively charged amino acids. From the cytoplasm, amino acids enter the circulation via selective channels in the basolateral membrane, and are carried to the circulation.

Lipids

Unlike carbohydrates and proteins, which are water soluble and therefore easily accessible to digestive enzymes and membrane transporters, lipids require partition into a hydrophobic or **amphipathic** environment. Churning and mixing and the **alkaline pH** of intestinal fluid promotes the formation of an **emulsion**.

Furthermore, **bile salts**, **phospholipids** and **cholesterol esters**, which are **amphipathic**, help to form **mixed micelles** with emulsified dietary lipids. These macromolecular complexes, in which amphipathic components create a hydrophobic core and a more hydrophilic, charged surface, carry digested lipids to the enterocyte surface.

The main dietary lipids are **triglycerides**, comprising three fatty acyl chains covalently linked to a glycerol backbone, **phospholipids**, in which one fatty acyl chain is replaced by a hydrophilic molecule, and **cholesterol esters**. **Lipases**, **phospholipases** and **cholesterol esterases**, the most important of which are synthesized by the pancreas, break down dietary lipids to fatty acids, monoacyl glycerol, lysophospholipids and cholesterol.

These digested lipids are absorbed across the cell membrane into the enterocyte cytoplasm where they are **re-esterified** and complexed with proteins called **apolipoproteins** to form lipid-rich lipoprotein particles known as **chylomicrons**.

Chylomicrons are actively secreted into the basolateral space and carried via lymphatic channels in the core of each villus, called **lacteals**, which carry them to the circulation via the thoracic duct. After a fatty meal, lacteals are filled with a milky, chylomicron-rich suspension.

Common disorders

The inability to digest and absorb macronutrients rapidly leads to **wasting** of muscle and fat. Eventually essential tissues such as skin, heart and epithelia cannot be maintained and patients die from **multiorgan failure**. These changes are also seen in **starvation**; however, if the cause is not reduced intake, but incomplete digestion and malabsorption, **diarrhoea**, **bloating** and **steatorrhoea** (passing fat-laden stool) also occur.

The commonest serious causes of macronutrient malabsorption are **coeliac disease**, which damages the intestinal mucosa, and **chronic pancreatitis**, which leads to pancreatic enzyme deficiency.

Other abnormalities of macronutrient absorption are relatively rare, except for **selective lactase deficiency**, which is genetically determined and very frequent in some ethnic groups, and may transiently may develop following a bout of infectious **gastroenteritis**. **Genetic** abnormalities of specific **transporters** cause deficiencies of specific amino acids. Genetic deficiency of **apolipoprotein B**, which is an essential component of chylomicrons, causes lipid deficiency and accumulation in enterocytes, which in turn causes general malabsorption.

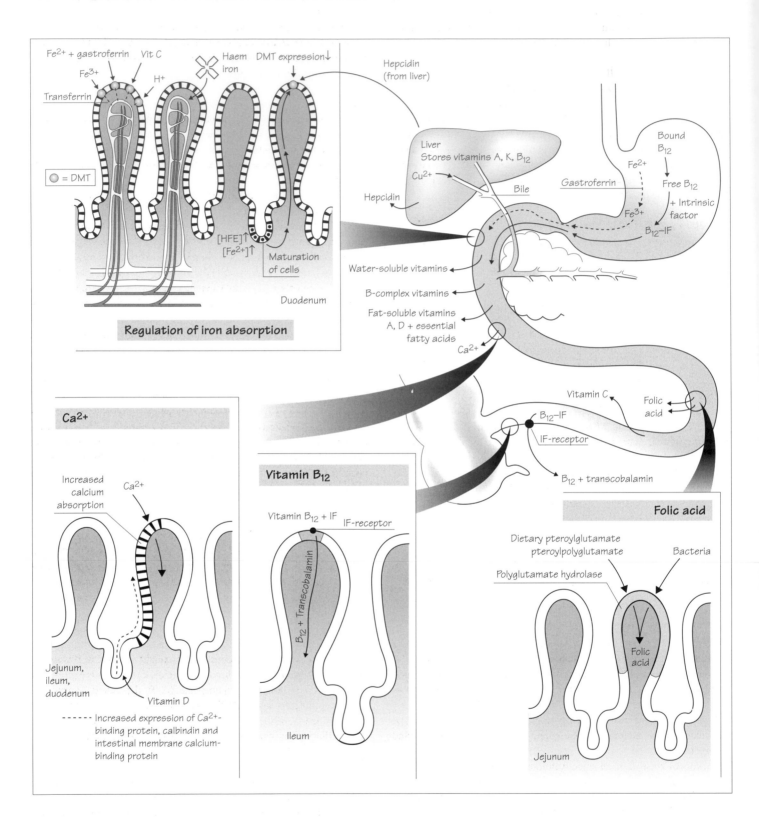

Fe^{2+} + gastroferrin Vit C

Transferrin

Fe^{3+} Fe^{2+} H$^+$ Haem iron DMT expression↓

= DMT

[HFE]↑
[Fe^{2+}]↑

Maturation of cells

Duodenum

Regulation of iron absorption

Hepcidin (from liver)

Liver
Stores vitamins A, K, B$_{12}$

Cu^{2+}

Hepcidin

Bile

Gastroferrin

Bound B$_{12}$

Fe^{2+}

Free B$_{12}$
+ Intrinsic factor

Fe^{3+}

B$_{12}$–IF

Water-soluble vitamins

B-complex vitamins

Fat-soluble vitamins
A, D + essential fatty acids

Ca^{2+}

Vitamin C Folic acid

B$_{12}$–IF

IF-receptor

B$_{12}$ + transcobalamin

Ca^{2+}

Increased calcium absorption Ca^{2+}

Jejunum, ileum, duodenum

Vitamin D

- - - - Increased expression of Ca^{2+}-binding protein, calbindin and intestinal membrane calcium-binding protein

Vitamin B$_{12}$

Vitamin B$_{12}$ + IF IF-receptor

B$_{12}$ + Transcobalamin

Ileum

Folic acid

Dietary pteroylglutamate pteroylpolyglutamate Bacteria

Polyglutamate hydrolase

Folic acid

Jejunum

Vitamins and minerals are essential dietary elements that are required in relatively small quantities and are known as **micronutrients**. Some are scarce and special adaptations help to garner the maximum amount from the diet. Some are potentially toxic and special mechanisms regulate their absorption, accumulation and excretion.

Water-soluble vitamins

The main water-soluble vitamins are **vitamin C** (ascorbic acid) and the **B-complex** vitamins. Ascorbic acid, thiamine (vitamin B_1), riboflavin, niacin, pyridoxine, biotin, pantothenic acid, inositol and choline are absorbed by passive diffusion or Na^+-dependent active transport in the small intestine. Vitamin C deficiency interferes with collagen synthesis and causes **scurvy**. B-complex vitamins are mainly involved in **energy metabolism** and deficiencies cause widespread abnormalities in epithelial, neuronal and cardiac function.

Vitamin B_{12} (hydroxocobalamin)

Dietary vitamin B_{12} is complexed with proteins that are degraded in the stomach. Vitamin B_{12} then binds to **intrinsic factor** (IF), a glycoprotein synthesized by gastric epithelial **parietal cells**. Intrinsic factor protects vitamin B_{12} from degradation in the intestine and binds to a receptor expressed on ileal enterocytes, which allows the complex to dissociate, so that the vitamin can be absorbed. In the circulation, absorbed vitamin B_{12} is transported bound to another protein, **transcobalamin**.

At least 3 months reserve of vitamin B_{12} is usually **stored** in the liver. Vitamin B_{12} is mainly derived from meat, eggs and milk, with little in vegetarian foods. **Vegans** are therefore particularly at risk of deficiency. Vitamin B_{12} deficiency may also be caused by gastric pathology, such as **atrophic gastritis**, where IF is not synthesized, or terminal ileal disease, such as **Crohn's disease**, where the absorptive surface is damaged. The **Schilling test** can distinguish between these causes (see Chapter 46).

Folic acid (pteroylmonoglutamate)

Folic acid is mainly derived from green leafy plants but may also be synthesized by intestinal bacteria. Folic acid and pteroylpolyglutamates are absorbed in the jejunum, where enterocytes cleave the polyglutamates to monoglutamates.

Folic acid and vitamin B_{12} are required for methylation reactions and deficiency has widespread effects, although the first observed clinical effect is usually **anaemia**, with enlarged, **megaloblastic** red cells.

Fat-soluble vitamins and essential fatty acids

Absorption of the **fat-soluble vitamins A**, **D**, **E** and **K** depends on adequate bile salt secretion and an intact small intestinal mucosa. Deficiencies therefore occur in **liver** disease, obstructive **jaundice** and **pancreatic** insufficiency, and with small intestinal pathology, such as coeliac disease.

Vitamin A (**retinoic acid**) is essential for many cellular functions and is critically important for vision. Deficiency causes **night-blindness** and dermatitis.

Vitamin D is essential for calcium homeostasis and healthy **bone formation**. Deficiency causes **osteomalacia** and **rickets**.

Vitamin E is an antioxidant and its exact role is being investigated.

Vitamin K is required for the post-translational modification (γ-carboxylation) of clotting factors. Deficiency causes **coagulopathy**.

Vitamin A is stored in **Ito cells** in the liver and vitamin D and K are stored in **hepatocytes**. They are not efficiently excreted, so they can accumulate in toxic quantities and supplements should be prescribed cautiously.

Linoleic, γ-linoleic, linolenic and arachidonic acid are all essential **polyunsaturated fatty acids** that cannot be synthesized in the body and are required for the synthesis of myelin in nerve tissue and prostaglandin synthesis (arachidonic acid).

Iron

Iron is an essential component of haemoglobin and other haem-containing proteins. **Iron deficiency** is a worldwide health problem causing **anaemia**, particularly in women of childbearing age. Conversely, excess iron is harmful and sophisticated mechanisms control its absorption.

Iron in haem (mainly derived from eating meat) is rapidly absorbed in the duodenum and is the most bio-available form.

Free dietary iron is usually present as **ferrous** (Fe^{2+}) or **ferric** (Fe^{3+}) iron. Ferric iron is not absorbed. Stomach acid and reducing agents, such as vitamin C, promote the conversion of Fe^{3+} to Fe^{2+} iron and absorption is therefore maximal in the acidic environment of the proximal duodenum. **Gastroferrin**, a glycoprotein secreted by gastric parietal cells, binds Fe^{2+}, preventing its binding to anions and maintaining its availability for absorption.

Iron is absorbed via the **divalent metal transporter** (DMT) protein in enterocytes. Absorbed iron leaves the basolateral membrane where it binds to circulating **transferrin**.

Excess body iron stores reduce iron absorption partly through decreased DMT expression. The **HFE protein**, expressed in immature intestinal cells, may act as an iron sensor, reducing DMT expression, and a circulating liver-derived peptide, **hepcidin**, also reduces intestinal iron absorption. **HFE** mutations in **hereditory haemochromatosis** cause uncontrolled iron absorption, which accumulates in the liver, pancreas, heart and other tissues and can cause liver cirrhosis, diabetes mellitus and cardiomyopathy.

Calcium

Calcium absorption occurs throughout the small intestine and is regulated by **vitamin D**, which stimulates the synthesis of calcium binding and transporting proteins in enterocytes, including the **intestinal membrane calcium-binding protein** and intracellular **calbindin**. Vitamin D deficiency therefore causes calcium deficiency, resulting in **osteomalacia** and **rickets**.

Copper

Copper is an essential cofactor for many oxidative enzymes. It is stored in the liver, bound to copper-binding proteins, and excess is excreted in the bile by an adenosine triphosphate (ATP)-dependent transporter, which is mutated in **Wilson's disease**, causing hepatic and neurological damage due to copper accumulation. Excess copper may also accumulate in biliary diseases such as primary biliary cirrhosis (**PBC**).

Zinc

Zinc is an essential cofactor in many enzymes and transcription factors and supplementation improves childhood resistance to gastroenteritis, suggesting that it plays a role in **immunity**. Zinc deficiency causes skin and intestinal abnormalities, including inclusions in Paneth cells, in a syndrome called **acrodermatitis enteropathica**.

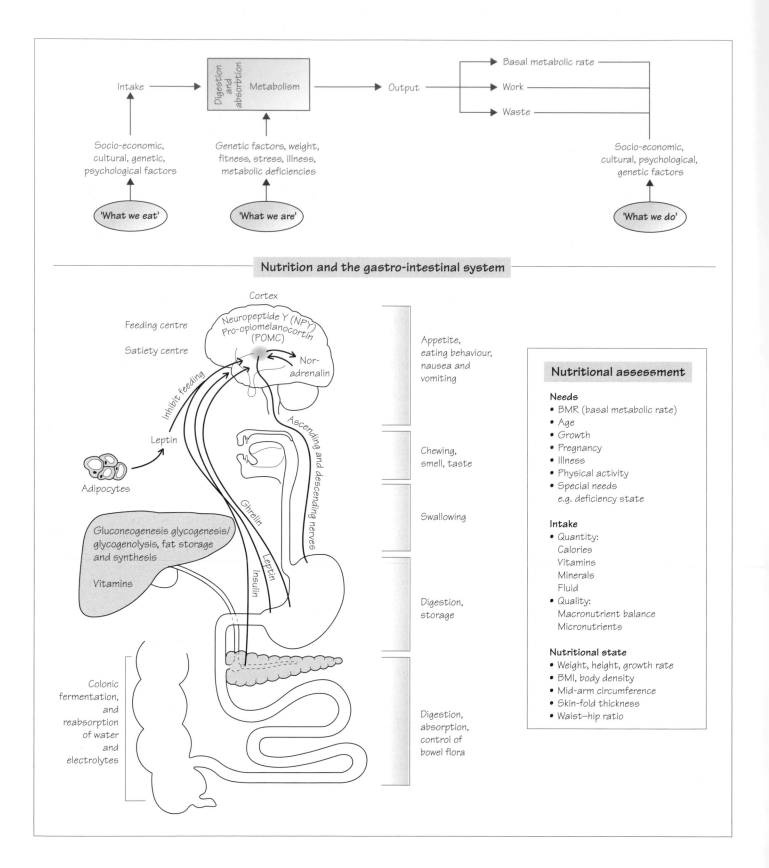

Nutrition and the gastro-intestinal system

Nutritional assessment

Needs
- BMR (basal metabolic rate)
- Age
- Growth
- Pregnancy
- Illness
- Physical activity
- Special needs
  e.g. deficiency state

Intake
- Quantity:
  Calories
  Vitamins
  Minerals
  Fluid
- Quality:
  Macronutrient balance
  Micronutrients

Nutritional state
- Weight, height, growth rate
- BMI, body density
- Mid-arm circumference
- Skin-fold thickness
- Waist–hip ratio

Assimilating nutrients is the central function of the gastrointestinal system, which also regulates their distribution, storage and disposal. Consequently, gastrointestinal dysfunction causes disordered nutrition and disordered nutrition has profound effects on the gastrointestinal system.

The slogan: 'what we eat, what we are and what we do' encapsulates nutrition. An adequate supply of nutrients must be available, the recipient must be in a state to metabolize nutrients to build and repair tissues and utilize chemical energy, and what ultimate use is made of nutrients is determined by what the recipient does.

Thus, a sedentary office worker uses food differently to an Olympic athlete or a critically ill patient on a mechanical ventilator. In each case what they do is potentially enhanced or limited by nutrition.

Basic nutritional concepts

The main foods, protein, carbohydrate and fat, are **macronutrients**, required in relatively large quantities to provide energy and organic building materials. **Micronutrients** are required in milligram or microgram quantities for special biochemical functions; these are mainly vitamins, minerals and essential fatty acids. Non-digestible plant material, called fibre or roughage, is needed for optimal intestinal function.

Energy intake must at least equal output. Even in a state of total rest, energy is required for metabolism—the **basal energy expenditure** (BEE). Basal energy expenditure varies with age and sex and most people must consume $1.3–1.5 \times$ their BEE to remain in equilibrium, although this may increase to $2 \times$ BEE with severe metabolic stress.

Metabolic energy is stored in the **chemical bonds** in organic compounds, with fats being the most **energy dense**, with the highest number of calories per gram weight, followed by carbohydrates and then proteins.

Glucose is essential for energy supply to the brain and red blood cells. It is usually derived from ingested polysaccharides, and the liver can maintain blood glucose levels from stored glycogen (**glycogenolysis**) and by converting amino acids to glucose (**gluconeogenesis**).

Although fats cannot be converted into glucose, metabolic adaptation in starvation means that the brain can use fatty acids and **ketones** for some of its energy requirements.

Amino acids are required to produce proteins, which are constantly renewed and replaced, even in adulthood when growth has ceased. Amino acid flux is measured in terms of **nitrogen balance**, as dietary nitrogen is almost entirely contained in amino acids and nitrogen excretion, via urea, is mainly due to amino acid breakdown. The dietary protein requirement to remain in nitrogen balance varies with **age**, **sex** and **metabolic state**.

Assessing nutrition

In children, **growth charts** help to detect potential nutritional problems. Other simple clinical measures include the **body mass index** (BMI) (weight/height^2), measured in kilograms and metres, giving a global measure, **mid-arm circumference**, reflecting muscle mass, and **skinfold thickness**, reflecting body fat.

Simple **blood tests** can identify deficiencies in iron, calcium, zinc, copper, vitamins A, D, K, B_{12} and folate, and nitrogen balance can be estimated by measuring urinary **urea** excretion.

Control of body mass

Maintaining healthy body weight and proportion through life is a complex feat of **neural and endocrine control**, the details of which are only now being discovered.

Food and calorie **intake** is regulated **behaviourally** and neuronal control involves the cortex and centres in the hypothalamus and brainstem. Many **neurotransmitters**, including peptide Y (PY), pro-opiomelanocortin (POMC), noradrenaline (NA) and serotonin (5-hydroxytryptamine, 5HT), are involved in the control of appetite. POMC- and PY-containing hypothalamic neurons integrate signals and communicate with the brainstem, which in turns signals to the hypothalamus using NA.

Leptin is a critically important peptide hormone released by **adipocytes** and **intestinal cells** to signal that adequate calories have been consumed and stored as fat. **Ghrelin**, released from the intestine, mediates long-term control of eating and body mass.

Body mass can also be controlled by regulating **energy expenditure**. In rodents, the basal metabolic rate (**BMR**) is increased by **adaptive thermogenesis**, whereby energy expenditure is increased in brown fat, generating heat. Humans have little brown fat, although BMR rises with regular exercise, which may explain how regular exercise improves weight control. However, BMR falls as body weight decreases, counteracting slimmers' efforts to lose weight.

Gastrointestinal disease and nutrition

Gastrointestinal disease inevitably interferes with nutrition. Reduced intake may be due to nausea and vomiting, poor dentition, or dysphagia secondary to oesophageal disease. Pancreatic, biliary and intestinal diseases cause **malabsorption**. Coeliac disease and Crohn's disease in particular are associated with multiple deficiencies, including calcium and vitamin D deficiency leading to osteoporosis.

Chronic liver disease is characterized by nutritional abnormalities and wasting of muscle and fat, while cholestatic liver disease reduces absorption of fats and fat-soluble vitamins.

Gastrointestinal diseases can also cause specific nutrient deficiencies, such as atrophic gastritis causing vitamin B_{12} deficiency.

Metabolic derangement caused by systemic disease is aggravated when the intestine, liver or pancreas is involved, as the patient's ability to assimilate nutrients is compromised.

Enteral and parenteral nutrition

High calorie liquid diets that can be administered by intravenous infusion have made **total parenteral nutrition** (TPN) possible. Total parenteral nutrition is used when patients cannot be fed enterally, for example, because of intestinal failure, or surgery.

With TPN, homeostatic mechanisms regulating digestion and absorption are bypassed; therefore, nutrient levels must be carefully monitored and the feed modified accordingly. This, and the risk of infection associated with infusing nutrient-rich solutions, make TPN demanding and potentially dangerous.

Furthermore, the lack of **enteral feeding** atrophies the intestinal epithelium and may increase bacterial translocation and the risk of sepsis. Thus, enteral or partial enteral nutrition is preferred.

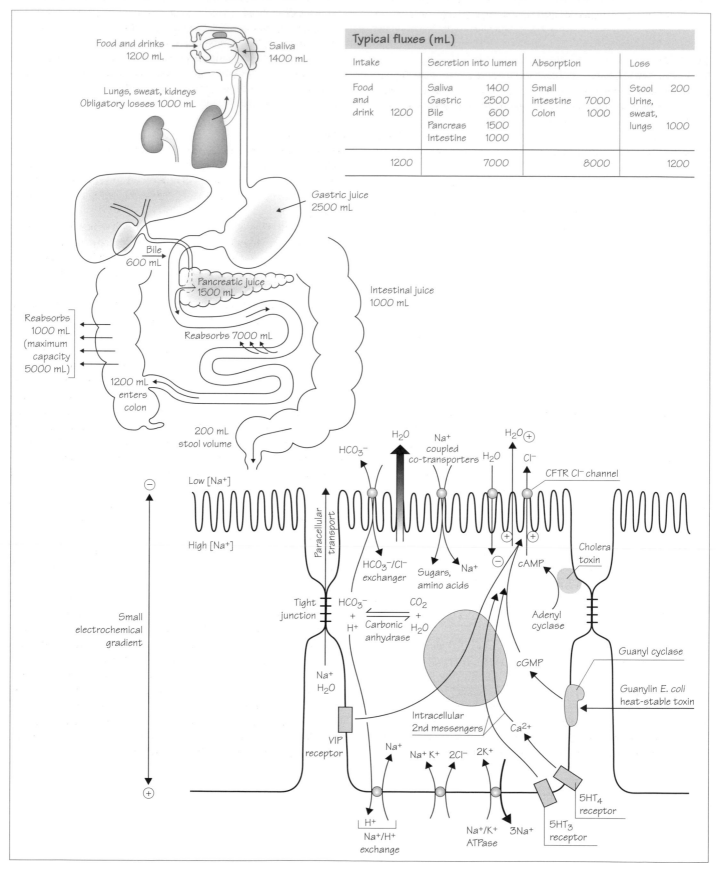

Food and drinks 1200 mL

Saliva 1400 mL

Lungs, sweat, kidneys Obligatory losses 1000 mL

Gastric juice 2500 mL

Bile 600 mL

Pancreatic juice 1500 mL

Intestinal juice 1000 mL

Reabsorbs 1000 mL (maximum capacity 5000 mL)

Reabsorbs 7000 mL

1200 mL enters colon

200 mL stool volume

Typical fluxes (mL)							
Intake		Secretion into lumen		Absorption		Loss	
Food and drink	1200	Saliva Gastric Bile Pancreas Intestine	1400 2500 600 1500 1000	Small intestine Colon	7000 1000	Stool Urine, sweat, lungs	200 1000
	1200		7000		8000		1200

Low [Na⁺]

H_2O

Na^+ coupled co-transporters H_2O

H_2O ⊕

Cl^-

HCO_3^-

CFTR Cl⁻ channel

High [Na⁺]

Paracellular transport

HCO_3^-/Cl^- exchanger

Sugars, amino acids

Na^+

⊕ ⊕

⊖ cAMP

Cholera toxin

Tight junction

HCO_3^- $+$ H^+

CO_2 $+$ H_2O

Carbonic anhydrase

Adenyl cyclase

Small electrochemical gradient

Na^+ H_2O

cGMP

Guanyl cyclase

Guanylin E. coli heat-stable toxin

Intracellular 2nd messengers

Ca^{2+}

VIP receptor

Na^+

Na^+ K^+ $2Cl^-$ $2K^+$

5HT₄ receptor

H^+ Na^+/H^+ exchange

Na^+/K^+ ATPase $3Na^+$

5HT₃ receptor

Body fluids and electrolytes must be replenished daily to make up for **obligatory losses** in sweat, urine, faeces and through the lungs. These amount to at least 1000 mL of water per day and are replaced by absorption in the intestine. Actual fluid fluxes are much larger, as exocrine glands secrete digestive juices that are reabsorbed distally.

Fluid flux

Typical fluid movements in the intact intestine are shown in the Figure.

The **small intestine** has a great capacity to secrete and absorb fluid under the **regulation** of enteric endocrine and neural signals and modified by bacterial and viral toxins, and drugs.

The **colon** can absorb up to 5000 mL of water per day, although inflammation, toxins and drugs can reduce this capacity. Small increases in fluid volumes reaching the colon can be compensated for by increased absorption; however, watery diarrhoea occurs when the amount of fluid leaving the terminal ileum exceeds colonic reabsorptive capacity.

Osmotically active substances in the small or large intestine, such as non-digestible or non-absorbable sugars, can overwhelm the ability of the small or large intestine to reabsorb water, causing diarrhoea.

Mechanisms

The intestinal lining comprises a single layer of **polarized epithelial cells** joined by **tight junctions**, effectively separating the luminal surface from the basolateral surface. Most fluid and electrolytes must therefore cross the epithelial cells, which maintain **gradients** and regulate fluxes through specialized **pores**, **channels** and **ion pumps** in their basolateral and apical membranes. There is also some **paracellular** movement of fluid and electrolytes, as tight junctions are not totally impermeable and their permeability can be altered by disease.

Water passively follows **osmotic gradients** generated by the secretion and absorption of ions and other osmotically active molecules. Apart from diet-derived small molecules, the main osmotic substances are Na^+, Cl^- and HCO_3^- ions. Also, K^+ is secreted along with Cl^- and HCO_3^- and, because body stores are relatively small, they can be severely depleted through intestinal losses.

The basolaterally situated $3 : 2$ **Na^+/K^+ ATPase pump** plays a major role in maintaining electrochemical gradients in enterocytes. It pumps two K^+ ions into the cell in exchange for three Na^+ ions out and thus depletes the enterocyte of Na^+ and maintains a **small negative electric potential** within the cell. Luminal Na^+ can then be transported into the enterocyte through selective pores and channels, along with, for example, monosaccharides and amino acids. Water passively follows these osmotically active ions.

In the ileum, caecum and distal large intestine, **Na^+ channels** allow Na^+ absorption independent of any co-transport, enabling further water reabsorption.

Cl^- secretion is mainly driven by a basolateral **$2Cl^-/Na^+/K^+$ transporter** that imports Cl^- into the cell. Regulated apical Cl^- channels, including the **cystic fibrosis transmembrane regulator** (CFTR), enable Cl^- efflux from the enterocyte along its electrochemical gradient. Intracellular cyclic adenosine $3',5'$-cyclic monophosphate (**cAMP**) lev-

els regulate the opening of CFTR, while other Cl^- channels are regulated by cyclic guanosine monophosphate (**cGMP**).

HCO_3^- secretion is important for maintaining alkaline pH of secretions in the salivary glands, small intestine, pancreas and biliary canaliculus. In the stomach, HCO_3^- secretion into the mucus layer buffers secreted HCl, protecting surface epithelial cells. HCO_3^- secretion is achieved by a combination of a basolateral **Na^+/H^+ exchanger** that transports H^+ out of the enterocyte, cytoplasmic **carbonic anhydrase**, which generates HCO_3^- and H^+ from CO_2 and H_2O, and an apical **HCO_3^-/Cl^- exchanger**.

Regulation

Dehydration is poorly tolerated and losing more than a few percent of body water results in fatigue, weakness, hypotension and circulatory failure. **Hypothalamic centres** that sense blood pressure and plasma osmolality, and use **vasopressin** as a neurotransmitter, control thirst and drinking.

A dry mouth also contributes to the sense of **thirst**; however, drinking rapidly satisfies subjective thirst, even if total body water is not replenished. Hydration should therefore be carefully evaluated and maintained in people who cannot eat and drink freely, such as critically ill patients.

Secretion is modified by many stimuli, including enteric hormones, inflammatory cytokines, bacterial and viral toxins and drugs. **Prostaglandins**, including synthetic misoprostol, used to counteract the ulcerogenic effects of non-steroidal anti-inflammatory drugs (NSAIDs) cause increased intestinal secretion. **Vasoactive intestinal peptide** (VIP) also enhances secretion, and VIP-secreting tumours cause the syndrome of watery diarrhoea and hypokalaemia. Serotonin (5-hydroxytryptamine, **5HT**) can increase or decrease secretion, depending on whether it acts on **$5HT_3$ or $5HT_4$ receptors**. **Somatostatin** inhibits intestinal secretion, partly by inhibiting the secretion of other enteric hormones. **Opioids** inhibit intestinal secretion and may promote **reabsorption** by reducing intestinal motility, which contribute to their antidiarrhoeal effect.

The main intracellular regulators of secretion and absorption are **cAMP**, **cGMP** and **Ca^{2+}**, which stimulates protein kinase C and its associated intracellular signalling pathways.

Certain **bacterial toxins** have well-characterized effects that illustrate how intestinal secretion is regulated. Cholera toxin B binds to cell surface receptors (GM1 ganglioside) facilitating the intracellular entry of **cholera toxin A**. Toxin A then irreversibly activates adenyl cyclase, generating excess **cAMP**. This stimulates Cl^- secretion through CFTR, which is followed by K^+ and Na^+ to maintain electroneutrality, and water along the osmotic gradient. The result is profound **secretory diarrhoea** that can cause life-threatening dehydration within hours.

The **heat-stable enterotoxin** (STa) of *Escherichia coli* stimulates receptors on the enterocyte surface that have **guanyl cyclase** activity and intracellular cGMP levels rise as a result. This stimulates Cl^- secretion, causing secretory diarrhoea similar to that caused by cholera toxin. The physiological role of **guanylin**, which is the natural, endogenous ligand for the receptor used by *E. coli* (STa), is still unknown.

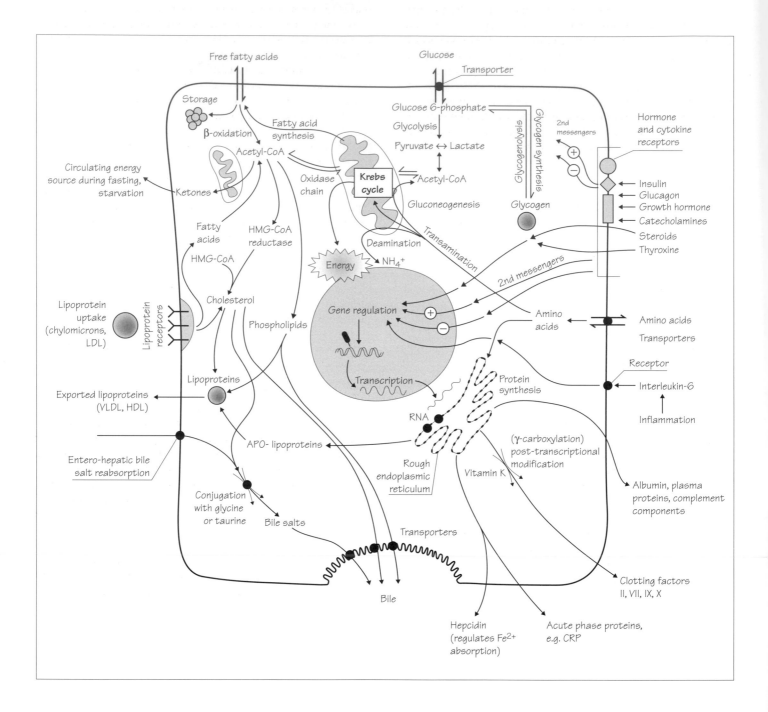

The liver is the metabolic powerhouse of the body, processing and controlling the daily inflow of nutrients from the digestive tract to maintain **homeostasis**. Biochemical pathways in the liver are internally integrated and externally controlled by hormones, growth factors and cytokines. The complexity of hepatic metabolic function is such that so far no totally artificial liver support device to replace the failing liver has been created.

Carbohydrates

Blood glucose levels are maintained within tight limits. Glucose is

essential for neuronal function and, if levels fall too low, **hypoglycaemia** causes **neuroglycopenia**, which can cause coma and death. On the other hand, sustained high blood glucose levels cause widespread damage to the body, particularly to blood vessels, as in diabetes mellitus.

The liver plays a critical role in maintaining normal blood glucose levels. It is a major store of glucose, in the form of **glycogen**, which is synthesized when there is excess substrate. The liver can store enough glycogen to be broken down by **glycogenolysis**, to maintain normoglycaemia for about 18 h. Athletes sometimes maximize liver glycogen stores before a competition by eating a carbohydrate-rich meal (**carbo-loading**).

The liver also produces glucose from **amino acids** by **gluconeogenesis**, whereby **transaminases** remove the amine group and feed the products into the **Krebs cycle**. Fatty acid metabolism also produces the two-carbon-containing acetyl coenzyme A (acetyl-CoA) molecule that feeds into the Krebs cycle; however, new six-carbon sugars, such as glucose, cannot be synthesized from fatty acids via the Krebs cycle. Thus sugar can be laid down as fat, but fat cannot be converted to sugar.

Hormones such as **insulin**, **glucagons**, **growth hormone**, **corticosteroids** and **catecholamines**, acting via cell-surface and intracellular receptors in the hepatocyte, determine the balance of glycogen synthesis, glycogenolysis and gluconeogenesis.

Lipids

Dietary lipids carried, for example, in chylomicrons, are taken up from the circulation by the liver and broken down into component parts including fatty acids, phospholipids and cholesterol.

The liver then repackages these lipids as **lipoproteins,** for export to the rest of the body via the bloodstream. Lipoproteins are macromolecular complexes formed from lipids and specific proteins called **apolipoproteins**. They allow hydrophobic lipids to be transported in the blood, and specific receptors that bind to different apolipoproteins allow targeting to the different tissues that express the necessary receptors. The main lipoproteins exported from the hepatocyte are **very low-density lipoproteins** (VLDL) and **high-density lipoproteins** (HDL).

The liver also takes up and recycles lipoproteins and free fatty acids from the circulation, further regulating the distribution of lipids around the body.

The liver is the major site of **cholesterol synthesis** and most circulating cholesterol is derived from hepatic synthesis rather than directly from the diet. The **statin** drugs, which are the most effective treatment for **hypercholesterolaemia**, act primarily on the liver, by inhibiting the rate-limiting enzyme in cholesterol synthesis, **HMG-CoA reductase**.

Cholesterol is used to synthesis **bile salts**, which are then conjugated with taurine and glycine (amino acids) and secreted in bile.

Ketones are synthesized from acetyl-CoA, derived from the oxidation of fatty acids and provide a source of circulating metabolic fuel during fasting and starvation. Cells such as neurons, which normally require glucose, can adapt their metabolism to use ketones.

Amino acids and proteins

Essential amino acids cannot be synthesized in sufficient amounts from precursors and must be derived from the diet. The liver produces a full complement of amino acids by **transamination** and other modifications of dietary amino acids and exports these for use in protein synthesis throughout the body.

Excess amino acids are metabolized by removal of the amino groups, releasing **ammonia**, which is potentially toxic and is converted into urea in the liver, via the **urea cycle**, and excreted in the urine. The carbon skeletons are used for energy production or converted into glucose for storage or export. Thus, during fasting, starvation or severe illness, the liver can convert muscle protein and other tissues into essential energy.

The liver synthesizes many proteins, including enzymes for its own metabolic processes, and **plasma proteins for export**. The liver produces **albumin**, which constitutes 50% of plasma protein, **coagulation factors** (including II, VII, IX and X, which are post-translationally modified by **vitamin K**-dependent **γ-carboxylation**) **complement** proteins, circulating **protease inhibitors**, **apolipoproteins** and **carrier proteins** that bind hormones and other small molecules in the circulation.

Inflammation causes the release of circulating peptide mediators called **cytokines**, of which interleukin 6 (**IL-6**), is particularly important in stimulating the hepatic **acute phase response**, whereby the liver rapidly increases its synthesis of host defence proteins and reduces albumin synthesis. Acute phase proteins include C-reactive protein (**CRP**), **serum amyloid A**, secretory phospholipase A2 and coagulation and complement proteins.

Metabolic and synthetic failure

All hepatocytes can perform basic metabolic and synthetic functions, so there is a vast **reserve capacity**. Disrupted carbohydrate, protein and lipid metabolism results in **fatigue**, **wasting** of body muscle and fat reserves, and biochemical abnormalities including **hypoglycaemia**, **hypoalbuminaemia** and reduced **coagulation factors**.

Hypoalbuminaemia can cause **oedema**, due to reduced plasma oncotic pressure allowing extravasation of fluid from capillaries into tissues. Reduced clotting factors cause a **coagulopathy**, with a prolonged **prothrombin time** (PT).

Coagulation factors have a half-life of few hours in the circulation and rapidly disappear when the liver fails suddenly. Albumin has a half-life of about 21 days, so it takes longer for levels to fall. Thus, the PT is the most sensitive clinical test of rapidly deteriorating liver function.

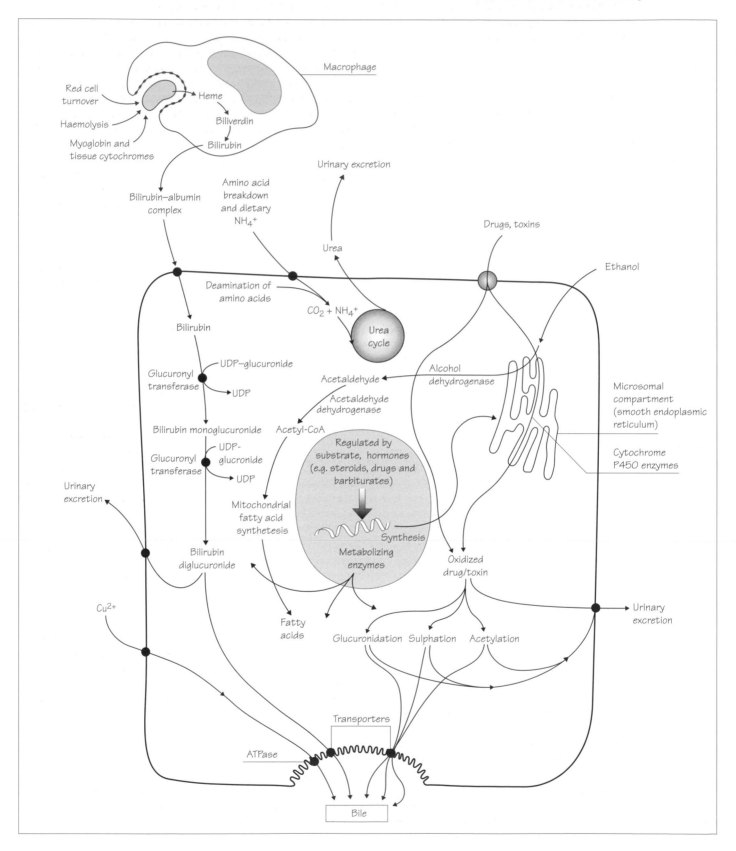

The liver has an immense capacity to metabolize biomolecules, inactivating them in most cases, and preparing them for excretion in bile or urine. Bilirubin metabolism typifies this and jaundice caused by impaired bilirubin excretion is a time-honoured marker of liver or biliary disease. The liver metabolizes many drugs and they should be cautiously prescribed to patients with impaired liver function.

Conjugation

Conjugating enzymes and their cofactors in the hepatocyte covalently link drugs, toxins and waste products with water-soluble moieties, such as **glucuronate**, **sulphate** and **alkyl** groups. The conjugated products are generally more **water-soluble** and are excreted either in the bile, via specific and general **transporters**, or in the urine, via the bloodstream.

Oxidases and cytochrome P450

The **smooth endoplasmic reticulum**, or microsomal compartment of the hepatocyte contains a large family of **oxidizing enzymes** linked to the cytochrome P450 proteins. These inactivate compounds by sequential oxidation, often rendering intermediates more water-soluble as well. Paradoxically, oxidation can increase the toxicity of a molecule, or may be required to activate the beneficial effect of a drug. Oxidized products are excreted in the bile or urine, or further conjugated.

Canalicular secretion

Conjugated molecules and certain essential **micronutrients**, which are potentially toxic, are excreted by hepatocytes into the bile. For example, **copper** is excreted by an adenosine triphosphate (ATP)-dependent transporter that is mutated in **Wilson's disease**, causing copper accumulation in the liver and in the central nervous system.

Urea cycle

Ammonia, generated by the metabolism of **amino acids**, is conjugated with CO_2 in a series of enzymatic reactions known as the urea cycle, generating urea, which is efficiently excreted in the **urine**.

Rare inherited defects in urea cycle enzymes cause **hyperammonaemia** and neurological dysfunction. Urea cycle activity is also reduced in severe liver disease and, when this occurs rapidly, as in **fulminant liver failure**, hyperammonaemia can cause **acute hepatic encephalopathy**, resulting in severe neurological damage, with incoordination, drowsiness, coma, and death due to cerebral oedema.

In chronic liver disease other factors, including toxins absorbed from the intestine, contribute to chronic hepatic encephalopathy.

The laxative **lactulose**, which is widely used to treat encephalopathy, **acidifies** the stool and limits ammonia absorption by ionizing it to non-absorbable ammonium ions.

Bilirubin

Bilirubin is a yellow-green **pigment** derived from the breakdown of **haem**, which is the oxygen-binding component of **haemoglobin, myoglobin** and **cytochromes**. Senescent red blood cells are ingested by macrophages, primarily in the spleen, and released haem is oxidized to **biliverdin** and then to bilirubin. Bilirubin is transported in the bloodstream bound to **albumin** and taken up by hepatocytes, where it binds to cytoplasmic proteins including glutathione S-transferase.

Bilirubin is conjugated with glucuronic acid by **glucuronyl transferase**, first forming bilirubin monoglucuronide, and then **diglucuronide**, which are more **water-soluble**. Some conjugated bilirubin

diffuses into the bloodstream and is excreted in the urine. Thus, there is normally some conjugated, and a much smaller amount of unconjugated, circulating bilirubin. Most conjugated bilirubin in hepatocytes is excreted into bile by **canalicular secretion**.

Unconjugated hyperbilirubinaemia may be caused by increased bilirubin production, as in **haemolytic disorders** (**prehepatic jaundice**). Liver disease seldom causes unconjugated hyperbilirubinaemia as there is a large reserve capacity of conjugating enzymes. However, a common inherited defect in the glucuronyl transferase enzyme can cause mild, fluctuating jaundice (**Gilbert's syndrome**) and no other abnormalities. In contrast, **Criggler–Najjar** syndrome, which is caused by a structural defect in the same gene, causes severe neonatal jaundice and neurological damage.

Conjugated hyperbilirubinaemia may be caused by **biliary obstruction** (**post-hepatic jaundice**). It may also be caused by liver disease affecting hepatocyte function, such as hepatitis, which interferes with transport protein function. This is called **intrahepatic cholestasis** (hepatic jaundice), as there is no macroscopic obstruction in the extrahepatic biliary system. Typically both conjugated and unconjugated bilirubin concentrations are increased.

Rarely, inherited defects in transport proteins cause conjugated hyperbilirubinaemia, as in the **Dubin–Johnson** and **Rotor syndromes**.

Alcohol (ethanol)

Alcohol, the most widely used psychoactive drug, is primarily metabolized in the liver. It diffuses freely into hepatocytes and is oxidized to **acetaldehyde** by the **alcohol dehydrogenase** enzyme. Acetaldehyde is extremely reactive, causing brain, liver and heart damage. It is inactivated by the enzyme **aldehyde dehydrogenase**, generating acetyl coenzyme A (acetyl-CoA), which can be converted into energy or stored as fat.

Inhibitors of aldehyde dehydrogenase, such as **disulfiram**, produce violent symptoms of intoxication if taken concurrently with ethanol and can be used to help people give up alcohol. Aldehyde dehydrogenase activity may be congenitally deficient, for example, in many Japanese people, who therefore are particularly sensitive to alcohol.

Paracetamol (acetaminophen)

Paracetamol is a potent cause of **fulminant liver failure** when taken in accidental or deliberate **overdose**. Paracetamol is normally mainly detoxified by **conjugation** with glucuronide. A small proportion is also oxidized by **microsomal oxidases**, forming a toxic metabolite, *N*-acetyl-*p*-benzoquinone-imine (NAPQI), which is then inactivated by conjugation with sulphate, derived from **glutathione**. However, in overdose, conjugation is saturated and a large amount of NAPQI is generated, which exhausts the liver's capacity for sulphation. NAPQI damages hepatocytes, further reducing the ability to neutralize the toxin. If administered soon enough, an antidote, *N*-acetylcysteine, which replenishes hepatic glutathione stores by donating sulphate groups, may prevent liver failure.

Regulation

Levels of detoxifying enzymes are regulated and, in some cases, for example with alcohol, regularly providing more **substrate** induces increased synthesis of the corresponding enzymes. **Drugs**, such as **steroid** hormones, **barbiturates** and certain **antiepileptics**, also induce the synthesis of hepatic enzymes. This is one mechanism by which drugs may interact, enhancing or diminishing each other's actions.

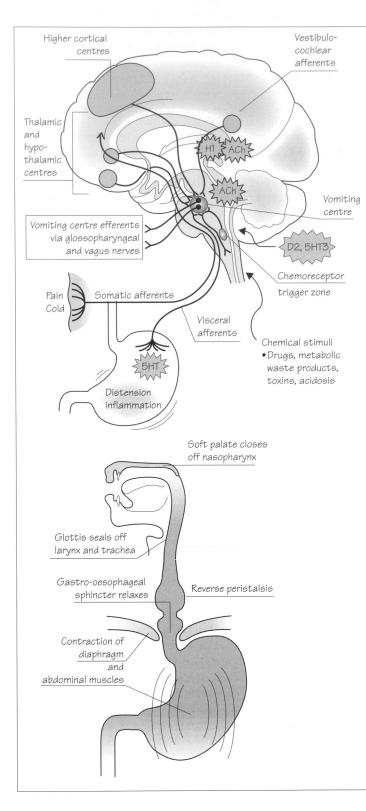

Higher cortical centres

Vestibulo-cochlear afferents

Thalamic and hypo-thalamic centres

H1 ACh

ACh

Vomiting centre

Vomiting centre efferents via glossopharyngeal and vagus nerves

D2, 5HT3

Chemoreceptor trigger zone

Pain Cold

Somatic afferents

Visceral afferents

Chemical stimuli
• Drugs, metabolic waste products, toxins, acidosis

5HT

Distension inflammation

Soft palate closes off nasopharynx

Glottis seals off larynx and trachea

Gastro-oesophageal sphincter relaxes

Reverse peristalsis

Contraction of diaphragm and abdominal muscles

Causes of vomiting

Cause	Mechanism
Motion sickness, vertigo, diseases of the ear	Vestibulocochlear inputs on vomiting centre (VC)
Intracranial pathology such as meningitis, raised intracranial pressure, migraine	Cortical and subcortical centre inputs on VC
Strong emotions, 'disgusting' sights, pain	Cortical inputs on VC
Drugs and chemicals, e.g. opiates, alcohol	Chemoreceptor trigger zone (CTZ) inputs on VC
Drugs that irritate the intestinal tract, e.g. chemotherapeutic agents for cancer	Vagal and autonomic inputs on VC
Gastrointestinal infections, food poisoning, appendicitis, cholecystitis	Vagal and autonomic inputs on VC, some emetogenic toxins directly stimulate VC
Intestinal obstruction, and distension	Vagal and autonomic inputs on VC
Systemic illness: diabetic ketoacidosis, ureamia, etc.	CTZ
Pregnancy	Hormonal changes including secretion of human chorionic gonadotrophin (βHCG)
Bulimia, voluntary emesis	Various pathways, including vagal afferents stimulated via the oropharynx (gag reflex)

Neurotransmitters and drugs

Drug	Neurotrasmitter receptor	Target
Hyoscine	Acetylcholine (ACh)	Vestibulocochlear nuclei, vomiting centre (VC)
Cyclizine	Histamine H1	Vestibulocochlear nuclei
Metoclopramide, prochlorperazine	Dopamine D2	Chemoreceptor trigger zone (CTZ)
Ondansetron	Serotonin (5HT3)	CTZ, gastrointestinal tract afferents

Forcefully expelling luminal contents from the stomach and intestine is an important defence against noxious agents that could be swallowed with food, and the process is tightly controlled. Vomiting is coordinated by signals from the intestine, body and brain, reaching nerve centres in the brainstem, which control voluntary and involuntary muscles in the abdomen, chest and gastrointestinal and respiratory tracts.

Nausea is the dysphoric desire to vomit, often accompanied by distaste for food and loss of appetite (anorexia). Although nausea usually precedes vomiting, either may occur in isolation.

Retching is the rhythmic reverse peristaltic activity of the stomach and oesophagus, accompanied by contraction of abdominal muscles and deep, sighing respiratory movements that often precede actual vomiting. Retching is 'dry', i.e. while it feels as though one is about to vomit, there is no efflux of vomitus. During retching, the oesophagus dilates and may accumulate vomitus that is subsequently expelled.

Vomiting is the forceful expulsion of food out of the mouth, usually accompanied by increased **salivation**, **sweating** and **tachycardia**. Vomiting is different from passive regurgitation, where acid stomach contents and partly digested food reflux into the mouth.

Muscular coordination

Intrinsic muscles of the stomach and oesophagus relax the gastro-oesophageal **sphincter** and force gastric contents out of the stomach and oesophagus by **reverse peristalsis**. Vomitus rarely contains material from beyond the ileocaecal valve, although reverse peristalsis can convey intestinal contents all the way from the **ileum**.

Abdominal muscles, including the diaphragm, contract, greatly increasing intra-abdominal and intrathoracic **pressure**, thus helping to empty the upper gastrointestinal tract.

Simultaneously, the **epiglottis** shuts off the **larynx**, which is drawn forward and upwards by muscles in the jaw and neck. The soft palate is drawn upwards, closing off the **nasopharynx**. These coordinated muscular movements protect the **airway** as vomitus is expelled. In unconscious or inebriated individuals these protective mechanisms are disrupted and vomitus may be aspirated into the airway.

Neural control

The **vomiting centre** (VC), in the dorsal part of the reticular formation of the **medulla oblongata**, is the main site of neural control of vomiting. The VC is essential for vomiting, whatever the primary stimulus, as it receives and coordinates signals from a number of other centres and coordinates the output.

The **chemoreceptor trigger zone** (CTZ) in the floor of the **fourth ventricle** lies outside the **blood–brain barrier** and therefore senses blood-borne chemical stimuli that induce vomiting, such as drugs like morphine and digoxin. The CTZ in turn stimulates the VC to induce vomiting.

Motion sickness and diseases of the inner ear cause vomiting by sending nerve signals from the nucleus of the **vestibulocochlear** (VIIIth cranial) nerve to the VC, possibly via the CTZ.

Other areas of the brain, such as the **cortex**, **thalamus** and **hypothalamus**, also signal to the VC, mediating vomiting associated with, for example, pain, emotional upset, fever and serious physical illness. **Variability** in the way that these stimuli are processed may account for why some people vomit more readily than others.

Sensory inputs from the gastrointestinal tract and other viscera, carried by the vagal and splanchnic autonomic nerves, also stimulate the VC, so that gastrointestinal distension, infection and inflammation can all induce vomiting.

The autonomic centres regulating sweating, lacrimation, salivation and heart rate all lie close to the VC and these autonomic phenomena are all stimulated in the surge of neuronal activity that accompanies vomiting.

Common causes

Common causes are detailed in the figure. **Neurogenic** or **psychic** stimuli, **chemicals** and **mechanical** or chemical irritation of the **intestinal tract** itself may stimulate vomiting. In many instances the exact pathway remains unknown.

Effects and consequences

Physiologically, vomiting **expels noxious material** from the gastrointestinal tract. Normally, neuromuscular reflexes protect the respiratory tract, but in inebriated or unconscious individuals protective mechanisms may fail, allowing **aspiration** of vomitus, which can cause asphyxiation or chemical inflammation and bacterial infection of the lungs (**pneumonia**).

The strong propulsive forces generated during retching and vomiting can cause a tear in the oesophageal mucosa (**Mallory–Weiss tear**). This typically causes haematemesis (vomiting blood). Generally the tear is superficial and heals rapidly.

Chronic vomiting, as in bulimia, can cause **acid damage to the teeth** and gums. Furthermore, prolonged or profuse vomiting can **deplete fluid and electrolytes**, leading to dehydration and altered blood chemistry. Vomiting of gastric contents typically causes **hypokalaemia**, **hyponatraemia** and **metabolic alkalosis**, while loss of HCO_3^- in intestinal contents can cause **metabolic acidosis**.

Treatment

Vomiting should generally be viewed as a **protective mechanism** and attention should be focused on treating the **underlying cause**, while supportive measures for the patient should aim to replace fluid and electrolyte losses.

In other cases, however, nausea and vomiting are stimulated by minor events, or by an essential treatment, such as chemotherapy for cancer, and must be treated even while the inducing agent is present. Fortunately, powerful drugs that interrupt vomiting in different ways are available. These include **acetylcholine (ACh)** receptor antagonists and **histamine H1** receptor antagonists, which are particularly useful for motion sickness and vestibulocochlear dysfunction; **dopamine D2** receptor antagonists, such as phenothiazines and metoclopramide, that block stimuli from the CTZ; **serotonin** (5-hydroxytryptamine, **5HT**) **5HT$_3$** receptor antagonists, such as ondansetron, that block the VC and afferents from the gastrointestinal tract; and **cannabinoids**, whose mechanism of action is still unknown.

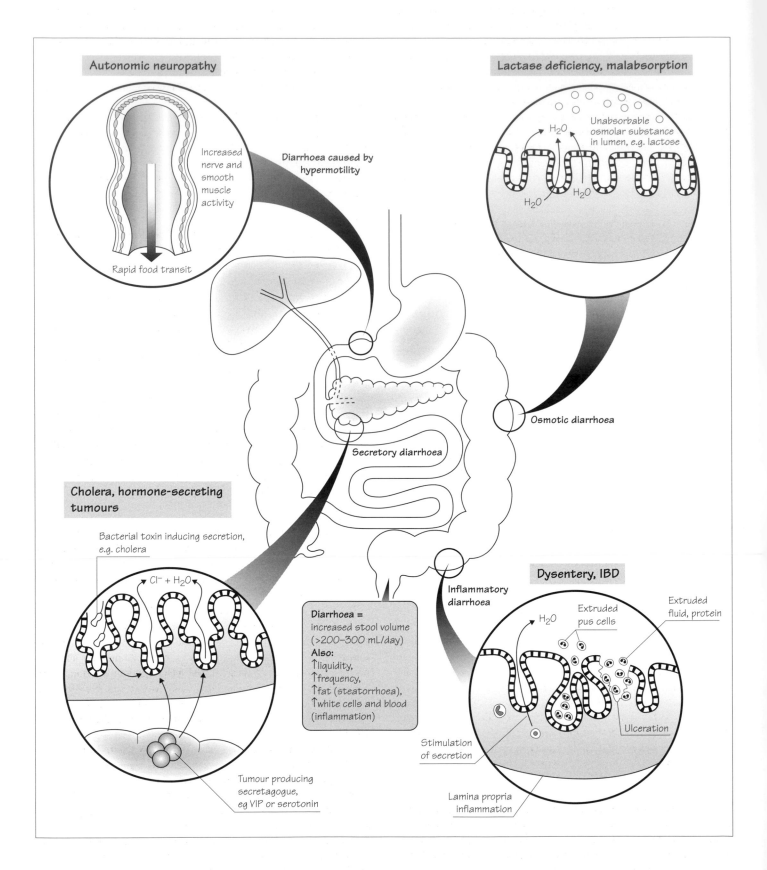

Autonomic neuropathy

Increased nerve and smooth muscle activity

Rapid food transit

Diarrhoea caused by hypermotility

Lactase deficiency, malabsorption

Unabsorbable osmolar substance in lumen, e.g. lactose

H_2O

H_2O

H_2O

Osmotic diarrhoea

Secretory diarrhoea

Cholera, hormone-secreting tumours

Bacterial toxin inducing secretion, e.g. cholera

$Cl^- + H_2O$

Tumour producing secretagogue, eg VIP or serotonin

Inflammatory diarrhoea

Diarrhoea =
increased stool volume
(>200–300 mL/day)
Also:
↑liquidity,
↑frequency,
↑fat (steatorrhoea),
↑white cells and blood
(inflammation)

Dysentery, IBD

H_2O

Extruded pus cells

Extruded fluid, protein

Ulceration

Stimulation of secretion

Lamina propria inflammation

Infectious diarrhoea is not only a nuisance to travellers—it also causes major morbidity and mortality in parts of the world where sanitation, clean drinking water and nutrition are inadequate. Diarrhoea can also be symptomatic of serious underlying gastrointestinal diseases, such as inflammatory bowel disease (IBD) and colorectal cancer.

By **definition**, diarrhoea implies that an **excess volume** of stool is passed, and this is usually accompanied by **increased frequency** of defecation and **increased liquidity** of the stool. Normal stool volume varies between individuals and is about 200–300 mL/day.

Diarrhoea may be accompanied by abdominal and rectal **pain**, **urgency** to defecate and **incontinence** of faeces. When diarrhoea is caused by food poisoning, there may be concurrent **vomiting**.

Diarrhoeal stool is usually more **liquid**. It may also contain more fat when caused by malabsorption (**steatorrhoea**) and it may contain **pus and blood** when caused by intestinal inflammation (see Chapters 34 & 35).

Diarrhoea is usually **acute**; that is, sudden in onset and short-lived, although it can be **chronic**. The causes, mechanisms and treatment are generally different in acute and chronic diarrhoea.

Mechanisms

Although the mechanisms are considered separately, for any one cause of diarrhoea multiple mechanisms may operate. For example, ulcerative colitis causes inflammation and also increased secretion and motility secondary to the stimulation of enteric neuro-endocrine pathways.

Secretory diarrhoea

When increased secretion into the intestine exceeds the capacity of the small and large intestine to reabsorb fluid, stool volume increases. Increased secretion by enterocytes is often aggravated by a concurrent absorptive defect.

Cholera is a common, serious and well-characterized example, where hypersecretion is mediated by the bacterial exotoxin of *Vibrio cholerae*. **Cholera toxin A** irreversibly activates **adenyl cyclase** to produce cyclic adenosine $3',5'$-cyclic monophosphate (**cAMP**), which stimulates sustained chloride secretion into the intestinal lumen by the cystic fibrosis transmembrane regulator (**CFTR**). Na^+ and water are secreted with Cl^-, maintaining electroneutrality and osmotic balance. Cholera can kill in a few hours by causing profound dehydration. The stool may be virtually clear electrolyte-rich fluid, known as '**rice-water stool**' (see Chapter 23).

Cholera is spread via the faecal–oral route, so diarrhoea enhances infectivity and aids the organism's survival. Conversely, diarrhoea clears bacteria from the intestine and is part of the body's defence system.

Other **bacterial toxins**, **hormones** elaborated by hormone-producing tumours, particularly **carcinoids** and vasoactive intestinal peptide (**VIP**)-omas, and **tubulovillous colonic adenomas** that secrete fluid and mucus from the abnormal epithelium can also cause secretory diarrhoea. Excess **bile salts** that are not reabsorbed in the terminal ileum, as a result of terminal ileal disease or resection, can induce colonic hypersecretion.

Osmotic diarrhoea

A **non-absorbable osmotic load** in the intestine can overload the intestine's capacity for reabsorbing water against the osmotic gradient. Thus more fluid remains in the intestinal lumen and is excreted, causing diarrhoea. An example is inherited or acquired **lactase deficiency**. Lactase is the enzyme that normally splits lactose, the predominant disaccharide in milk, into the absorbable monosaccharides glucose and galactose. Without lactase, ingested lactose remains in the intestine, creating an osmotic load. Hereditary lactase deficiency is more frequent in populations where milk is a minor part of the traditional diet, and can also be acquired as a result of damage to the intestinal epithelium, caused by, for example, **gastroenteritis**.

Other causes of osmotic diarrhoea include the use of non-absorbable **food sweeteners**, such as sorbitol, and **laxatives**, such as lactulose and magnesium sulphate.

Malabsorption of other dietary components can also cause diarrhoea, although generalized malabsorption, such as in pancreatic failure, predominantly causes **steatorrhoea**, which is increased **faecal fat** content, causing large, pale stools that float on water and have an unpleasant odour, partly due to metabolism of fatty acids by colonic bacteria.

Inflammation

Damage to the intestinal lining, caused by bacterial or viral **infection**, or **immune-mediated** processes, causes infiltration of fluid and inflammatory cells into the intestinal wall and extrusion of this inflammatory **exudate** into the intestinal lumen. Excess mucus may also be secreted by the damaged epithelium. Inflammation also increases fluid secretion and inhibits reabsorption (see Chapters 32 & 34).

Pain and **urgency** often accompany inflammatory diarrhoea and **leucocytes** and **blood** are found mixed in with the stool.

Common causes include bacterial and amoebic **dysentery** and **IBD**.

Dysmotility

Increased motility can increase the **frequency** of defecation, and when it is severe there may be insufficient time for normal **reabsorption** of fluid from the stool, resulting in increased stool volumes. Dysmotility may occur with **autonomic neuropathy**, for example, in diabetes mellitus. Other causes include **thyrotoxicosis** and motility-stimulating **drugs**, such as acetylcholinesterase inhibitors used to treat myasthenia gravis (see Chapters 15 & 17).

Treatment

Most acute diarrhoea is caused by **short-lived and self-limiting** bacterial or viral infection and, as the diarrhoea is a **defence mechanism** against infection, antidiarrhoeals should be used with caution. Treatment should be mainly supportive, to prevent dehydration and electrolyte depletion.

Hydration can be maintained using a slightly hypotonic and alkaline **oral rehydration solution** containing **glucose** and **sodium** in the correct ratio to exploit active absorption via the apical Na^+–glucose co-transporter on enterocytes, which draws water into the cells along the osmotic gradient (see Chapter 23). The WHO rehydration formulation is 3.5 g NaCl, 1.5 g KCl, 2.9 g Na citrate and 20 g glucose per litre. This provides 90 mM Na^+, 20 mM K^+, 80 mM Cl^-, 10 mM citrate and 111 mM glucose. In more severely ill patients **intravenous hydration** may be required.

Specific causes can also be treated, for example, **antibiotics** for bacterial or amoebic dysentery and **steroids and 5-aminosalicylates** for IBD. Malabsorption caused by pancreatic insufficiency can be treated with oral **pancreatic enzyme supplements**, while secretory diarrhoea caused by hormone-secreting tumours can be controlled using **somatostatin**, which reduces hormone secretion.

The most frequently used **antidiarrhoeals** are the **opiates** codeine and loperamide, which inhibit intestinal motility and increase the time available for intestinal fluid reabsorption.

28 Constipation

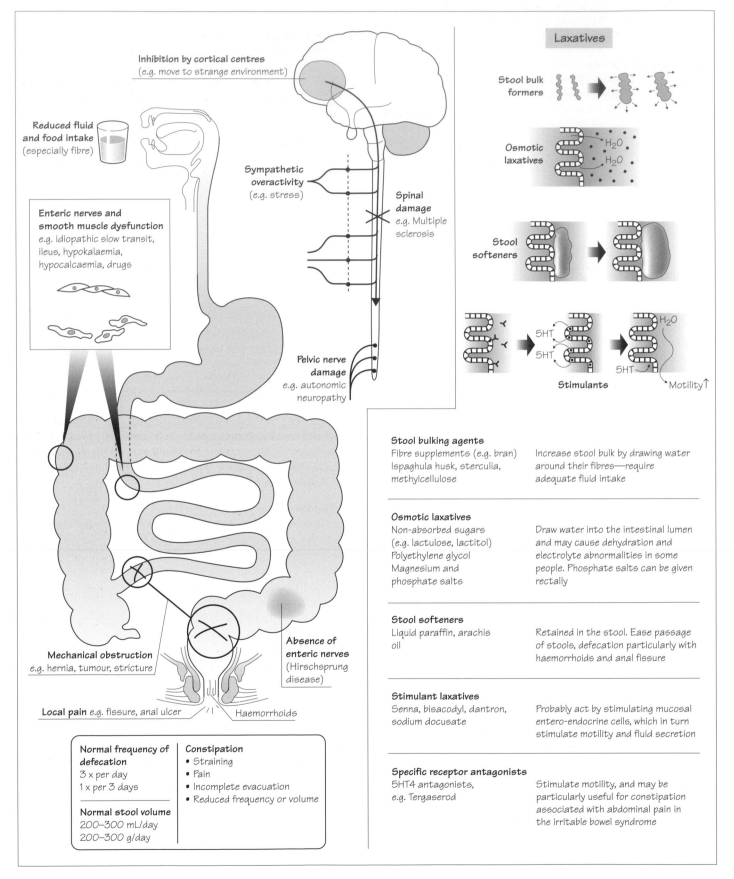

Inhibition by cortical centres
(e.g. move to strange environment)

Reduced fluid and food intake
(especially fibre)

Sympathetic overactivity
(e.g. stress)

Spinal damage
e.g. Multiple sclerosis

Enteric nerves and smooth muscle dysfunction
e.g. idiopathic slow transit, ileus, hypokalaemia, hypocalcaemia, drugs

Pelvic nerve damage
e.g. autonomic neuropathy

Mechanical obstruction
e.g. hernia, tumour, stricture

Absence of enteric nerves
(Hirschsprung disease)

Local pain e.g. fissure, anal ulcer

Haemorrhoids

Laxatives

Stool bulk formers

Osmotic laxatives H$_2$O H$_2$O

Stool softeners

Stimulants 5HT 5HT 5HT H$_2$O Motility↑

Normal frequency of defecation 3 x per day 1 x per 3 days	**Constipation** • Straining • Pain • Incomplete evacuation • Reduced frequency or volume
Normal stool volume 200–300 mL/day 200–300 g/day	

Stool bulking agents Fibre supplements (e.g. bran) Ispaghula husk, sterculia, methylcellulose	Increase stool bulk by drawing water around their fibres—require adequate fluid intake
Osmotic laxatives Non-absorbed sugars (e.g. lactulose, lactitol) Polyethylene glycol Magnesium and phosphate salts	Draw water into the intestinal lumen and may cause dehydration and electrolyte abnormalities in some people. Phosphate salts can be given rectally
Stool softeners Liquid paraffin, arachis oil	Retained in the stool. Ease passage of stools, defecation particularly with haemorrhoids and anal fissure
Stimulant laxatives Senna, bisacodyl, dantron, sodium docusate	Probably act by stimulating mucosal entero-endocrine cells, which in turn stimulate motility and fluid secretion
Specific receptor antagonists 5HT4 antagonists, e.g. Tergaserod	Stimulate motility, and may be particularly useful for constipation associated with abdominal pain in the irritable bowel syndrome

Constipation is one of the commonest gastrointestinal complaints. In addition, people often attribute symptoms such as tiredness, lethargy, nausea and headache to what they perceive as constipation. Often no medical explanation is found and there is no proven link between infrequent defecation and general ill health.

Causes and mechanisms

Irregular bowel habit can exacerbate constipation, as the colon and rectum continue to remove water from stool, hardening it and making passage more difficult. Thus, constipation can be **self-perpetuating**. In severe chronic constipation, particularly in the elderly, faeces may become so hard, dry and immovable (**faecal impaction**) that they cannot be passed without medical or surgical assistance, leading to intestinal obstruction.

Reduced motility

Reduced colonic motility may be congenital as in **Hirschsprung's disease**, where myenteric nerves are absent from the distal colon, causing chronic obstruction and a massively dilated, faeces-filled proximal colon (**megacolon**).

Paralytic ileus occurs after abdominal **surgery**, or with **electrolyte abnormalities**, such as hypokalaemia. Intestinal motility may be reduced acutely by **stress**, due to sympathetic autonomic nerve activity, and people who are severely injured or otherwise unwell may become constipated for several days.

Neuromuscular dysfunction caused by **hypercalcaemia** directly reduces intestinal motility.

Reduced colonic motility may also be **constitutive**, i.e. normal for that person (**slow transit constipation**).

Drugs

Drugs such as opiates, antidepressants and others with **anticholinergic** effects reduce intestinal motility. Similar effects are seen with oral iron supplements and aluminium-containing antacids.

Excessive, chronic use of **stimulant laxatives**, such as senna, can reduce motility, presumably by damaging or depleting enteric neurons, causing colonic atonia.

5HT$_3$ receptor antagonists that have been used to treat diarrhoea in irritable bowel syndrome (IBS) can also cause severe constipation.

Stool bulk

Stool volume and the frequency of defecation vary with diet, fluid intake and intestinal secretion. **Dietary fibre**, which mainly comprises non-digestible plant polysaccharides, draws **water** around itself, increasing stool volume. Thus, chronic constipation is often caused by lack of dietary fibre and/or **inadequate fluid intake**, which is required to hydrate dietary fibre and to soften the stool.

With **fasting**, the frequency of defecation declines, partly because of reduced reflex colonic activity and also because of reduced stool volume, although a large proportion of the solid material in stool actually comprises enteric bacteria rather than food residue.

Neuro-psychological dysfunction

Defecation is imbued with **social** and psychosexual **constraints** that influence bowel habit, and it can be inhibited **voluntarily** via the **external anal sphincter** and by **cortical signals** acting on autonomic nerves.

Neurological damage to the **brain and spinal cord**, for example, in **multiple sclerosis** and **peripheral neuropathy** can lead to chronic constipation as well as incontinence.

Local causes and obstruction

Local obstruction, for example, by a tumour, may cause pain and difficulty in defecation. Painful local lesions, such as **prolapsed haemorrhoids** and anal **fissure**, inhibit the urge to defecate. Constipation and straining at stool contributes to the development of haemorrhoids and fissure.

Clinical features

The **normal frequency** of defecation (bowel movement, bowel opening) **varies** in the population from around three times a day to once every 3 days, although many people lie outside this range.

Alteration of previously regular bowel habit is more likely to indicate disease, although some causes of constipation are congenital.

True constipation implies reduced defecation frequency or stool volume, although patients also complain of **straining** during defecation, **pain** on defecation and hard, dark stool. The sense of incomplete evacuation is called **tenesmus**.

Paradoxically, chronic constipation and faecal impaction, particularly in the elderly, may cause incontinence and passage of fluid per rectum, so-called **overflow incontinence**.

Diagnosis

Perceived and actual problems must be distinguished. A **careful history** of dietary habits and any drugs that might cause constipation should be taken.

Faecal impaction and local lesions, including anal and rectal cancer, can be detected by **digital rectal examination**. Faecal loading of the colon may be seen on plain abdominal X-ray. Timing the passage of radio-opaque markers through the intestine (**shape test**) is used to diagnose slow transit constipation.

Treatment

Stopping drugs that cause constipation and ensuring that sufficient **fibre** and **fluid** are ingested are essential. Increasing dietary fibre forms the basis of laxatives that rely on increasing stool bulk, although excess fibre can exacerbate constipation.

Where **psychological or social factors** are implicated, it is important that they are identified.

Correcting **electrolyte abnormalities** and allowing the bowel time to recover usually resolves paralytic ileus.

Mechanical obstruction and Hirschsprung's disease are treated **surgically**. Painful or obstructive peri-anal and rectal conditions may also require surgery.

Where constipation does not respond to simple dietary or lifestyle measures, and is not caused by identifiable pathology, **laxatives** may be used. They work in a number of different ways, including increasing **stool bulk**, increasing **osmotic** fluid secretion, **softening stool**, **stimulating** secretion and motility via enteric neuro-endocrine pathways and directly stimulating neuro-endocrine responses by **receptor-targeting**. These are detailed in the table within the figure opposite.

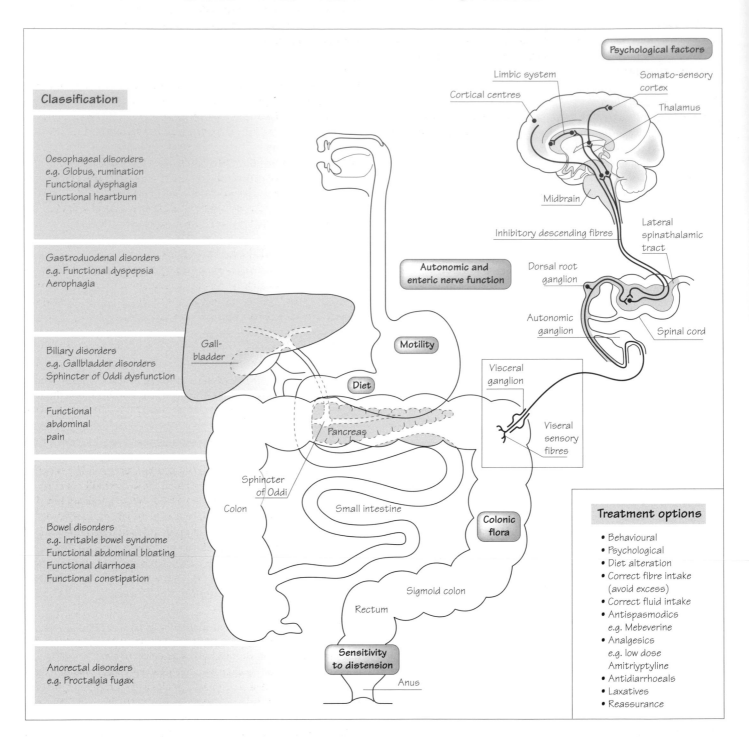

Classification

Oesophageal disorders
e.g. Globus, rumination
Functional dysphagia
Functional heartburn

Gastroduodenal disorders
e.g. Functional dyspepsia
Aerophagia

Biliary disorders
e.g. Gallbladder disorders
Sphincter of Oddi dysfunction

Functional
abdominal
pain

Bowel disorders
e.g. Irritable bowel syndrome
Functional abdominal bloating
Functional diarrhoea
Functional constipation

Anorectal disorders
e.g. Proctalgia fugax

Treatment options

- Behavioural
- Psychological
- Diet alteration
- Correct fibre intake
  (avoid excess)
- Correct fluid intake
- Antispasmodics
  e.g. Mebeverine
- Analgesics
  e.g. low dose
  Amitriyptyline
- Antidiarrhoeals
- Laxatives
- Reassurance

Gastrointestinal symptoms without discernable organic pathology are **common**, occurring in a quarter of the population and accounting for half of all consultations with gastroenterologists. Although many people have symptoms that are consistent with a clinical diagnosis of a functional bowel disorder, only a minority seek medical attention.

Although the symptoms can be distressing, these disorders do not predispose to more serious illness, so patients can be reassured once serious pathology has been excluded.

The pathogenesis of functional bowel disorders is unknown and their treatment remains unsatisfactory, but in some patients at least, symptoms can be partially relieved.

Definition

The basic feature of these disorders is pain or discomfort referred to the gastrointestinal tract, with some altered bowel function, such as diarrhoea or constipation. The diagnosis is **clinical**, based on patients in the right demographic group presenting with **typical symptoms** in the **absence of any evident pathology**. Symptoms are more likely to be due to functional bowel disorders in younger people and due to more serious disorders, such as cancer, in older people.

Classification

Discrete syndromes, classified according to the part of the gastrointestinal system affected, have been formally defined to assist diagnosis, treatment and research.

Oesophageal disorders

These include common conditions, such as **heartburn** without significant acid regurgitation, and rare syndromes, such as **globus hystericus**, where patients sense a lump in the throat.

Gastroduodenal disorders

Here symptoms mimic peptic ulcer disease, gastritis and other serious disorders, without any evident pathology. The commonest syndrome is **non-ulcer dyspepsia**.

Abdominal pain syndromes

Chronic abdominal pain can be very troublesome and when no obvious pathology accounts for the symptoms, the pain is classified as functional.

Irritable bowel syndrome

Many patients fall into this diagnostic group, with abdominal pain, bloating and altered intestinal function. Diarrhoea or constipation may predominate and both symptoms can occur in the same patient.

Formal diagnostic criteria are still being evolved and the original formal criteria established in the 1980s gives a sense of what irritable bowel syndrome (IBS) comprises of:
• At least 6 months of abdominal pain or discomfort, typically relieved by defecation, and two or more of the following:
  • altered stool frequency;
  • altered stool consistency;
  • altered stool passage (e.g. urgency, straining, incomplete evacuation);
  • passage of mucus;
  • abdominal bloating.

Biliary syndromes

The symptoms suggest biliary disease without any evidence of pathology. In some cases spasm of the **sphincter of Oddi** can be demonstrated.

Anorectal syndromes

Patients may complain of difficulty passing stool, or pain associated with defecation. Recurrent pain in the anal canal with no demonstrable organic pathology is known as **proctalgia fugax**. Excessive anal sphincter tension and sweating may lead to peri-anal itching (**pruritis ani**).

Pathophysiology

Numerous physiological alterations have been described that could account for some of the functional bowel disorder syndromes. Often, however, so-called abnormalities simply reflect extremes of normal function.

Increased visceral sensitivity

Experiments show, for instance, that patients with IBS experience pain on rectal distension more readily than do control subjects.

Cultural and psychological factors affect pain perception, partly through spinal gating of painful stimuli, whereby inhibitory neurons from cortical centres release endogenous opiates onto spinal interneurons that convey pain signals to the brain, and thus reduce the central transmission of pain.

Altered motility

Diarrhoea and constipation could result from altered intestinal transit time, but physiological studies of intestinal motility are still inconclusive. Altered function of smooth muscle in extra-intestinal organs, such as the lungs and urinary bladder has been demonstrated in IBS.

Altered autonomic and enteric nervous system function

Vagal and sympathetic dysfunction has been demonstrated in small numbers of patients. Increased activity of intrinsic enteric neurons, particularly those using **serotonin** (5-hydroxytryptamine, **5HT**), may account for altered motility and visceral hypersensitivity.

Diet, infection and altered bowel flora

Many patients report increased sensitivity to particular foods. Interactions between diet and the resident intestinal bacteria probably have significant effects on bowel function, but systematic studies and experimental data to support this are still lacking.

Psychological factors

Patients with functional bowel disorders generally score higher on **anxiety and depression questionnaires**, although cause, effect and simple association are hard to separate. Even if psychological factors do not cause symptoms, they may predispose people to seek medical attention.

Diagnosis

While avoiding excessive investigation, which increases the patient's anxiety that 'something must be wrong and the doctors still can't find it', some simple tests are usually performed to **exclude serious underlying pathology**. These include a blood count, serum electrolyte determination, serological tests for coeliac disease, gastro-oesophageal endoscopy, sigmoidoscopy or colonoscopy, and stool culture.

There are **no specific tests** for functional bowel disorders, although visceral sensitivity, intestinal motility and alterations in bowel flora are all being investigated experimentally.

Treatment

Establishing a firm diagnosis, excluding serious organic pathology and reassuring patients are the mainstay of treatment so far.

Dietary and lifestyle changes often help, especially avoiding excess alcohol and foods that precipitate symptoms, and regulating **dietary fibre** and **fluid** intake. Excess fibre can aggravate abdominal pain and bloating, while too little can contribute to chronic constipation.

Behavioural therapy including relaxation, hypnosis and biofeedback helps some patients, as does psychotherapy.

Symptomatic pharmacological treatment is appropriate. Thus **diarrhoea** may be treated with antidiarrhoeals, **constipation** with laxatives and **pain** with low doses of tricyclic antidepressants that reduce pain perception. Smooth muscle relaxants, or **antispasmodics** such as mebeverine and peppermint oil may relieve the pain associated with spasm and bloating. $5HT_3$ and $5HT_4$ receptor antagonists are being developed to target diarrhoea and constipation specifically.

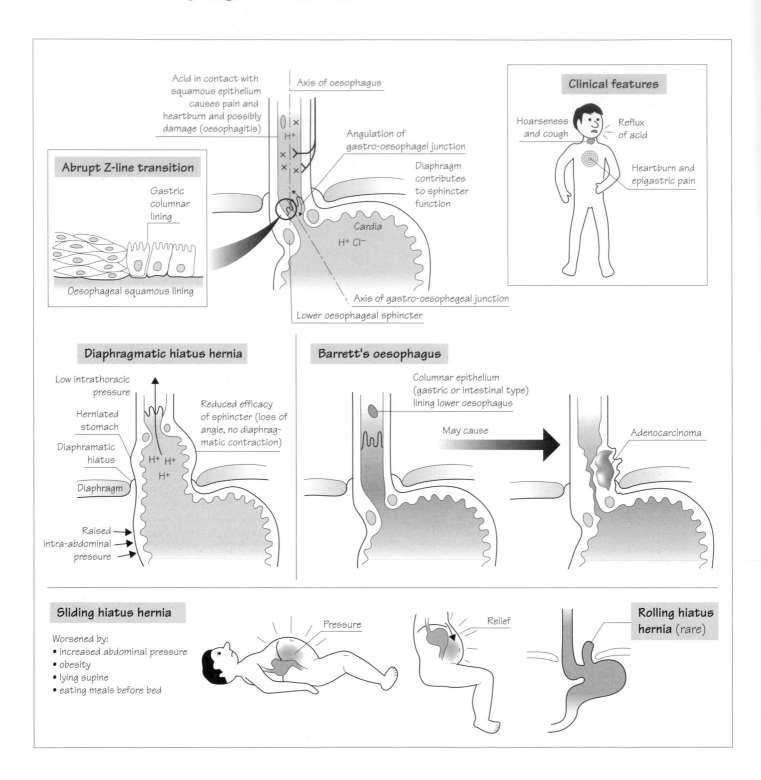

Abrupt Z-line transition

Acid in contact with squamous epithelium causes pain and heartburn and possibly damage (oesophagitis)

Axis of oesophagus

Angulation of gastro-oesophagel junction

Diaphragm contributes to sphincter function

Gastric columnar lining

Oesophageal squamous lining

Cardia
H⁺ Cl⁻

Axis of gastro-oesophegeal junction

Lower oesophageal sphincter

Clinical features

Hoarseness and cough

Reflux of acid

Heartburn and epigastric pain

Diaphragmatic hiatus hernia

Low intrathoracic pressure

Herniated stomach

Diaphramatic hiatus

Diaphragm

Raised intra-abdominal pressure

Reduced efficacy of sphincter (loss of angle, no diaphragmatic contraction)

H⁺ H⁺ H⁺

Barrett's oesophagus

Columnar epithelium (gastric or intestinal type) lining lower oesophagus

May cause

Adenocarcinoma

Sliding hiatus hernia

Worsened by:
• increased abdominal pressure
• obesity
• lying supine
• eating meals before bed

Pressure

Relief

Rolling hiatus hernia (rare)

Symptoms indicating possible gastro-oesophageal reflux are common in the general population. They vary greatly in severity and the actual underlying damage is also variable, so that careful and thorough diagnostic evaluation is needed to guide treatment.

Pathogenesis

Tonic contraction of thickened intrinsic **circular smooth** muscle closes off the gastro-oesophageal junction, separating the gastric and oesophageal lumens. **Diaphragmatic muscle fibres** reinforce this sphincter function and the oesophagus enters the gastric fundus at an **angle**, which also tends to seal the junction. Furthermore, while the lower oesophagus and gastro-oesophageal junction remain in the abdominal cavity, any increase in **intra-abdominal pressure**, which tends to squeeze gastric contents out of the stomach, also impinges on the junction and counteracts this effect.

Stomach contents do regularly reflux through the gastro-oesophageal sphincter, even in normal individuals, when the lower oesophageal sphincter relaxes to allow food, drink and swallowed saliva to enter the stomach. This physiological reflux is probably not harmful.

However, when oesophageal and diaphragmatic muscle tone declines and intra-abdominal pressure is chronically increased, for example, by obesity, particularly in older individuals, reflux may become more frequent and severe.

Reflux of gastric contents stimulates **nerve endings** in the lower oesophagus, which can cause pain and discomfort. Chronic stimulation may also increase the **sensitivity** of nerve endings, causing pain even in the absence of concurrent reflux. Severe and prolonged reflux can damage and erode the lower oesophageal epithelium and provoke inflammation (**oesophagitis**).

Chronic reflux can also induce metaplastic change in the epithelial lining of the lower oesophagus, which is normally a non-cornified stratified squamous epithelium, and can change to a simple columnar epithelium, with gastric or small intestinal features. This **gastric or intestinal metaplasia** is known as **Barrett's oesophagus**, which may undergo **dysplasia** and can go on to develop into **adenocarcinoma** (see Chapters 4 & 38).

The most likely cause of damage due to reflux is **gastric hydrochloric acid** (HCl), although other gastric contents, such as **enzymes**, and **bile acids** from the duodenum, may also contribute. Bile acids, chemically altered by acid, may be particularly important in inducing metaplasia, dysplasia and cancer.

Helicobacter pylori infection tends to reduce gastric acid secretion, particularly when it causes chronic gastritis, so that, theoretically, eradication of *H. pylori* infection, which reduces the risk of gastritis, peptic ulcer and gastric cancer, may actually exacerbate acid reflux (see Chapter 31).

Reflux can be further aggravated by the development of a **hiatus hernia**, which forms when part of the stomach herniates through the hiatus (or gap) in the diaphragm through which the oesophagus enters the abdomen. As a result, the herniated portion of the stomach comes to lie in the thorax. Usually the gastro-oesophageal junction and gastric cardia slide upwards, creating a **sliding hiatus hernia**, which compromises sphincter function by straightening out the angle of the gastro-oesophageal junction and removing the diaphragmatic contribution to sphincter function. Furthermore, as the junction now lies within the thorax, which has a low pressure, increased intra-abdominal pressure, transmitted through the stomach, tends to force gastric contents through the sphincter.

A sliding hiatus hernia can **spontaneously reduce**, for example, when lying flat, and by reducing intra-abdominal pressure, which encourages the stomach to return to the abdomen.

Less frequently, a fold of gastric cardia may herniate through the diaphragmatic hiatus alongside the oesophagus, creating a **rolling hiatus hernia**, which can become strangulated.

Clinical features

Heartburn is described by patients as an acid, burning sensation in the epigastrium or lower chest, often localized to just behind the sternum (retrosternally). It is the typical symptom of gastro-oesophageal reflux. Patients may also complain of **epigastric pain** and dyspepsia aggravated by meals, alcohol and lying flat in bed.

Stomach contents may reflux into the mouth and occasionally be aspirated into the larynx, causing **cough** and **hoarseness**. Reflux may also be completely **asymptomatic** and, paradoxically, the development of Barrett's oesophagus, which is relatively resistant to acid damage, may improve symptoms.

Diagnosis

Upper gastrointestinal **endoscopy** is the main diagnostic test. Biopsies are taken to distinguish oesophagitis and Barrett's oesophagus **histologically**. A **barium swallow** can demonstrate hiatus hernia and reflux of stomach contents into the oesophagus, as well as severe degrees of oesophagitis.

Oesophageal and gastric **pH** can be measured directly via a nasogastrically placed sensor. Episodes of reduce pH can then be correlated with symptoms and in the **Bernstein test**, acid is infused into the lower oesophagus, in an attempt to reproduce the symptoms and confirm the diagnosis (see Chapter 46).

Oesophageal manometry helps to distinguish dysmotility from reflux (see Chapter 46).

Treatment

Lifestyle changes such as having smaller meals, giving up smoking, reducing alcohol intake, losing weight and sleeping with the head of the bed raised can effectively reduce symptoms. Simple antacids are also effective, although selective histamine **H2 receptor antagonists**, such as **ranitidine**, and the **proton pump inhibitors**, such as **omeprazole**, which irreversibly block acid production by parietal cells, are the most effective treatment.

Hiatus hernia usually does not require specific treatment, such as **surgery**, although it can be repaired by **fundoplication**, whereby the gastric fundus is partially wrapped around the lower oesophagus, strengthening the sphincter and preventing migration through the diaphragmatic hiatus. Fundoplication can also be used to treat intractable reflux in the absence of a hiatus hernia.

Barrett's oesophagus is **premalignant** and, therefore, regular endoscopic **surveillance** with biopsies to detect dysplasia is advocated. If dysplasia is detected, the patient may undergo **oesophagectomy**.

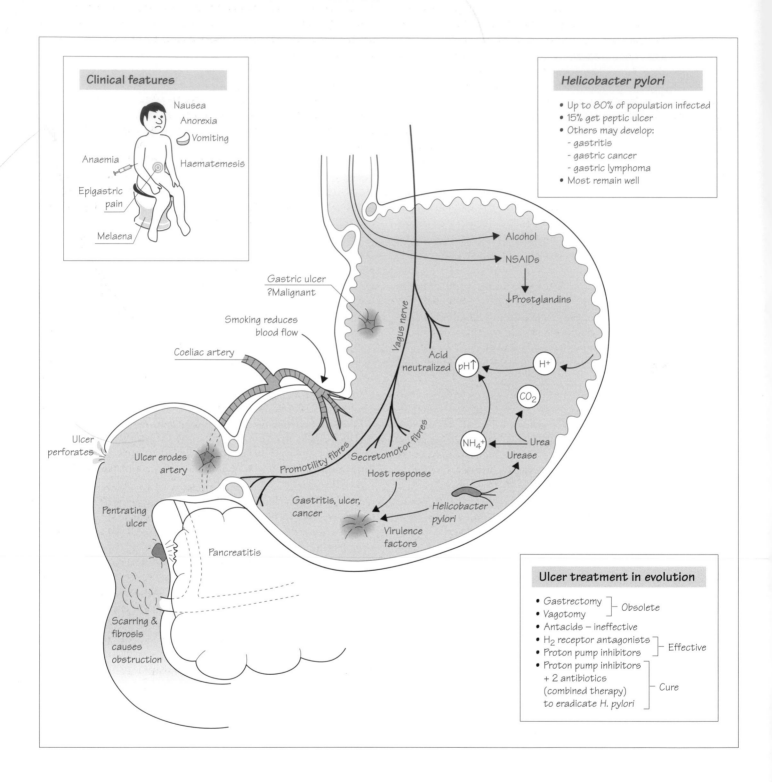

Clinical features

Nausea
Anorexia
Vomiting
Anaemia
Haematemesis
Epigastric pain
Melaena

Helicobacter pylori

- Up to 80% of population infected
- 15% get peptic ulcer
- Others may develop:
  - gastritis
  - gastric cancer
  - gastric lymphoma
- Most remain well

Gastric ulcer ?Malignant

Smoking reduces blood flow

Coeliac artery

Ulcer perforates

Ulcer erodes artery

Pentrating ulcer

Pancreatitis

Scarring & fibrosis causes obstruction

Vagus nerve

Promotility fibres

Secretomotor fibres

Host response

Gastritis, ulcer, cancer

Virulence factors

Alcohol

NSAIDs

↓Prostglandins

Acid neutralized

pH↑

H+

CO_2

NH_4^+

Urea

Urease

Helicobacter pylori

Ulcer treatment in evolution

- Gastrectomy
- Vagotomy ⎤ Obsolete
- Antacids – ineffective
- H₂ receptor antagonists
- Proton pump inhibitors ⎤ Effective
- Proton pump inhibitors + 2 antibiotics (combined therapy) to eradicate H. pylori ⎤ Cure

Peptic ulcers are common, affecting 15% of individuals in the Western world. In many cases they cause only mild symptoms and little damage, but in others they can be life threatening. The treatment of peptic ulcer has dramatically changed following our improved understanding of its pathogenesis, representing a triumph of the power of scientific medicine.

Pathology

The surface epithelium of the stomach or duodenum is damaged and ulcerates, and the resulting inflammation extends into the underlying mucosa and submucosa. Gastric **acid** and **digestive enzymes** penetrate into the tissues, causing further damage, for example, to blood vessels and adjacent tissues.

Pathogenesis

• **Acid**. Gastric acid (**HCl**) production is stimulated by **gastrin** secreted by G cells in the antrum, **acetylcholine** released by the vagus nerve and **histamine** released by entero-chromaffin-like (ECL) cells, all of which stimulate receptors on acid-producing **parietal cells**.

Duodenal ulcers are exceedingly rare in people who do not produce gastric acid and multiple, recurrent ulcers occur when acid production is greatly increased, for example, by gastrin-secreting tumours (see Chapters 16 & 38). However, gastric acid production is usually low in people with gastric ulcers and this may be the result of chronic gastritis.

• **Prostaglandins**. The risk of peptic ulcer is increased in patients who use non-steroidal anti-inflammatory drugs (**NSAIDs**), including aspirin, which inhibit prostaglandin production by epithelial cells. Furthermore the risk of peptic ulcer is reduced by an artificial prostaglandin E2 agonist, misoprostil.

• **Smoking, alcohol, genetics** and **stress**. Other risk factors include smoking tobacco and drinking alcohol, although the mechanisms by which these act are unknown. In addition, there is a small genetic predisposition. There is little evidence that stress or lifestyle factors play any role.

• *Helicobacter pylori*. Spiral bacteria in the stomach had been noted for over a hundred years, yet their significance only became apparent in 1982 when Warren and Marshall cultured *H. pylori* from 11 patients with gastritis and Dr Marshall then demonstrated that it caused gastritis by ingesting a test dose himself. He was subsequently cured by antibiotic treatment.

H. pylori infection is present in the majority of patients with peptic ulcer, although only about 15% of infected people develop ulcers. Eradicating *H. pylori* infection permanently cures peptic ulcer in the majority of cases.

H. pylori infection of the **gastric antrum**, which stimulates gastrin production, causes the greatest hyperacidity and **duodenal ulceration**, while infection of the **gastric corpus**, where most parietal cells are present, tends to reduce stomach acid production and is associated with **gastritis, gastric ulcer, gastric cancer** and **gastric lymphoma**.

Strains of *H. pylori* vary in **pathogenicity** and **virulence**, determined by various bacterial gene clusters. Thus both host factors and the bacterial strain determine the outcome of infection.

Peptic ulceration results from an imbalance between **gastroprotective** factors, such as the mucus layer and prostaglandins, and **aggressive factors**, such as stomach acid and the effects of smoking, alcohol and NSAIDs. *H. pylori* infection dramatically tips the balance against protection.

Clinical features

Epigastric pain, often aggravated by hunger or by meals and relieved by antacids, suggests peptic ulceration or gastritis. There may be nausea, vomiting and anorexia. **Anaemia** may develop from chronic haemorrhage.

Peptic ulcer may cause major acute bleeding, leading to **haematemesis** and/or **melaena**, which is a medical emergency. Similarly, peptic ulcers may perforate the stomach or duodenum, causing **peritonitis**. Peptic ulcer may **penetrate** into the pancreas and cause **pancreatitis**. Scarring of the duodenum by chronic ulceration may cause intestinal **obstruction**.

Diagnosis

Upper gastrointestinal **endoscopy** is the best diagnostic test. Ulcers can also be detected by **barium** contrast X-rays.

H. pylori infection can be diagnosed **serologically**, or by the **urease breath test**, in which ^{13}C-labelled urea is taken orally and the resulting $^{13}CO_2$ released by the urease enzyme is measured on the breath (see Chapter 46). *H. pylori* organisms can be demonstrated **histologically** and the urease enzyme can be detected using a simple colorimetric test (**CLO test**, for *Campylobacter*-like organism) in mucosal biopsies taken during endoscopy (see Chapter 46).

Gastric ulcers may be caused by **carcinoma** or **lymphoma**, so they must always be **biopsied** to check that they are not malignant. Duodenal ulcers are very rarely malignant.

Treatment

• **Surgery**. Except for emergencies, surgical treatment is now obsolete. **Partial gastrectomy** to remove part of the gastrin-producing, G-cell-rich antrum was once routinely performed. Another approach was to selectively section branches of the vagus nerve (**selective vagotomy**) that stimulated acid secretion, sparing fibres that controlled the pyloric sphincter.

• **Simple antacids** and **anticholinergics** are relatively ineffective, have to be taken frequently and produce side-effects.

• The first effective medical treatment for peptic ulcer emerged when selective histamine **H2 receptor antagonists** were developed. For some time drugs such as cimetidine and ranitidine were the most widely prescribed medications worldwide.

• **Proton pump inhibitors**, which irreversibly block acid production by parietal cells, have overtaken the H2 receptor antagonists, and **omeprazole**, the first proton pump inhibitor, accounts for the greatest worldwide expenditure on a single drug.

• *Helicobacter pylori* **eradication** provides a permanent cure for most cases of peptic ulcer. Successful eradication requires **combined therapy** with an acid suppressor and two or three antibiotics. Most standard regimes are successful in up to 90% of cases, although antibiotic resistance is emerging.

• **Emergency treatment**. Bleeding or perforation may require emergency **surgical** or **endoscopic** therapy, such as injection of adrenaline around an exposed vessel, to arrest haemorrhage.

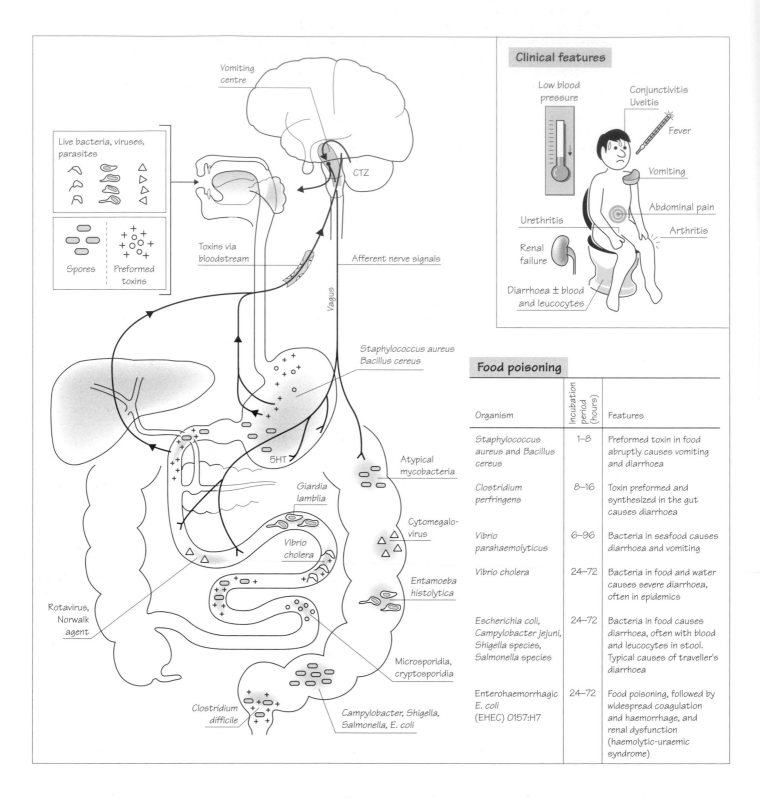

Live bacteria, viruses, parasites

Spores | Preformed toxins

Vomiting centre

CTZ

Toxins via bloodstream

Afferent nerve signals

Vagus

Staphylococcus aureus
Bacillus cereus

5HT

Atypical mycobacteria

Giardia lamblia

Cytomegalovirus

Vibrio cholera

Entamoeba histolytica

Rotavirus, Norwalk agent

Microsporidia, cryptosporidia

Clostridium difficile

Campylobacter, Shigella, Salmonella, E. coli

Clinical features

Low blood pressure

Conjunctivitis
Uveitis

Fever

Vomiting

Abdominal pain

Urethritis

Arthritis

Renal failure

Diarrhoea ± blood and leucocytes

Food poisoning

Organism	Incubation period (hours)	Features
Staphylococcus aureus and Bacillus cereus	1–8	Preformed toxin in food abruptly causes vomiting and diarrhoea
Clostridium perfringens	8–16	Toxin preformed and synthesized in the gut causes diarrhoea
Vibrio parahaemolyticus	6–96	Bacteria in seafood causes diarrhoea and vomiting
Vibrio cholera	24–72	Bacteria in food and water causes severe diarrhoea, often in epidemics
Escherichia coli, Campylobacter jejuni, Shigella species, Salmonella species	24–72	Bacteria in food causes diarrhoea, often with blood and leucocytes in stool. Typical causes of traveller's diarrhoea
Enterohaemorrhagic E. coli (EHEC) O157:H7	24–72	Food poisoning, followed by widespread coagulation and haemorrhage, and renal dysfunction (haemolytic-uraemic syndrome)

Gastroenteritis is common, causing illness ranging from self-limited episodes of food poisoning, experienced occasionally by most people, to devastating epidemics that cause many deaths worldwide. In addition, many systemic infections enter the body through the intestine. Viruses, bacteria, fungi, protozoa and multicellular parasites are all implicated.

Pathogenic mechanisms

Microorganisms cause gastroenteritis in a number of ways:
• **Enterotoxins**. These are usually secreted proteins that act on the intestinal epithelium, or are absorbed into the bloodstream and have systemic effects. For example, vibrios and enterotoxigenic *Escherichia coli*

(ETEC) secrete heat-sensitive or heat-stable enterotoxins that drive excessive intestinal secretion. *Staphylococcus aureus* and *Bacillus cereus* produce emetogenic toxins that are absorbed systemically and stimulate the vomiting centre. Some toxins cause intestinal inflammation; for example, the cytotoxin secreted by *Clostridium difficile*.

• **Adhesion and persistence in the intestine.** The flow of luminal contents through the intestine limits harmful microbial effects and some organisms overcome this defence mechanism by producing adhesive structures (**adhesins**) that interact with proteins on the host cell surface. Multicellular parasites, such as worms, may use mechanical hooks and suckers to resist being swept away.

• **Invasion of epithelial cells and mucosal damage.** Enteropathogenic *E. coli* (EPEC), *Campylobacter jejuni*, *Salmonella* and *Shigella* species, *Vibrio parahaemolyticus*, viruses such as cytomegalovirus, and amoebae (*Entamoeba histolytica*), invade the epithelium, causing ulceration and inflammation. In bacterial, viral and amoebic dysentery, the stools contain blood and leucocytes and there is a systemic inflammatory response, resembling inflammatory bowel disease.

• **Invasion through the intestine.** The dysentery-causing bacteria, *E. histolytica* and *Salmonella typhi*, the cause of typhoid fever, may cross the epithelium and cause local and distant disease. *S. typhi* initially multiplies in intestinal lymphoid tissue; however, the most serious effects of typhoid result from systemic bacteraemia. Invasion is an essential step in the lifecycle of some parasites and worms.

Clinical features
Typically infection rapidly follows ingestion of contaminated **food** or **drink** and is **short-lived** and **self-limiting**.

Vomiting may be induced directly by **emetogenic enterotoxins** and is also mediated by **efferent nerves** stimulated by intestinal distension and mucosal damage. Serotonin (5-hydroxytryptamine, **5HT**) released from neuro-endocrine cells may stimulate the chemoreceptor trigger zone (CTZ) (see Chapter 26).

Diarrhoea is caused by numerous factors: **toxins** stimulating secretion; **neuro-endocrine** reflexes stimulating motility and secretion; **inflammation** causing **exudation** of fluid and cells into the intestine; and a reduced digestive and absorptive capacity for sugars (particularly lactose), creating an **osmotic** load (see Chapter 27).

Abdominal pain is caused by **distension** of the intestine, muscle **spasms** resulting from hypermotility, and **inflammatory damage** to the mucosa.

Fever and other systemic symptoms are unusual with simple gastroenteritis or food poisoning, although they are frequent in bacterial or amoebic **dysentery**. They suggest invasive infection.

Dehydration may cause **hypotension** and **renal failure**.

Heamolytic–uraemic syndrome is a life-threatening syndrome caused by enterohaemorrhagic *E. coli* (EHEC) serotype 0157:H7, which is endemic among cattle. Outbreaks have often been traced to inadequately cooked **ground beef**. Vomiting and diarrhoea are followed by high fever and damage to blood vessels, and the kidneys may be damaged by the EHEC cytotoxin. Antibiotics may aggravate the syndrome.

Reiter's syndrome and other reactive arthritis syndromes, characterized by combinations of arthritis, urethritis, conjunctivits, uveitis and various mucocutaneous lesions may follow bacterial dysentery.

Guillain–Barré syndrome, caused by immune-mediated demyelination of peripheral nerves, may follow *Campylobacter* infection.

Gastroenteritis can also cause prolonged **lactose intolerance** and **post-infectious irritable bowel syndrome**.

Food poisoning
This is the common syndrome of gastroenteritis caused by contaminated food. Usually **spores** or **organisms** that multiply in the intestine are ingested. In cases where **preformed toxins** are ingested, symptoms occur sooner, within hours (see table within the figure).

Traveller's diarrhoea
Travellers to areas where gastrointestinal infection is common, typically Africa, the Far East and Latin America, are at risk. **Bacteria** like *Campylobacter*, *Shigella*, *Salmonella* and *E. coli* are the commonest cause, followed by **viruses** and **protozoa** (*Giardia lamblia* and *Entamoeba histolytica*).

Endemic and epidemic diarrhoea
Outbreaks of gastroenteritis occur in nurseries, schools, camps and hospitals where overcrowding and communal facilities allow rapid spread. Viruses such as the **rotavirus** and the **Norwalk** agent are the commonest cause. Wars, floods and earthquakes can create conditions for outbreaks of **cholera** and **typhoid**. These outbreaks, aggravated by scarcity of clean drinking water and basic medical care, can cause great suffering.

Immunocompromised patients
Diarrhoea is common and often chronic in patients with acquired immune deficiency syndrome (**AIDS**) and in those who are immunosuppressed. Organisms that are normally non-pathogenic, such as *Cryptosporidia* and **microsporidia**, can cause **opportunistic** disease.

Antibiotic-associated diarrhoea
Antibiotics alter the normal balance of enteric commensal bacteria and may cause diarrhoea. This is frequently caused by overgrowth of toxin-producing *Clostridium difficile*, which can cause severe inflammation (**pseudomembranous colitis**).

Diagnosis
Blood and **leucocytes in stool** distinguish inflammatory diarrhoea from other causes.

Microbiological diagnosis may be necessary for **public health** reasons, or to diagnose the cause of persistent diarrhoea. Rotavirus is detected in the stool by **electron microscopy** and amoebae can be detected by light microscopy. Bacterial pathogens require stool **culture**, while giardiasis requires **jejunal aspiration** and microscopy to make the diagnosis.

Treatment
The mainstay of treatment is to maintain hydration, either with **oral rehydration solutions** or **intravenous** fluids (see Chapters 23 & 27).

Antibiotics like **ciprofloxacin** can reduce the duration and severity of bacterial gastroenteritis but are usually unnecessary. Giardiasis and amoebiasis are effectively treated with **metronidazole**.

Because diarrhoea is a host defence mechanism against infection, antidiarrhoeals like **loperamide** should generally be avoided.

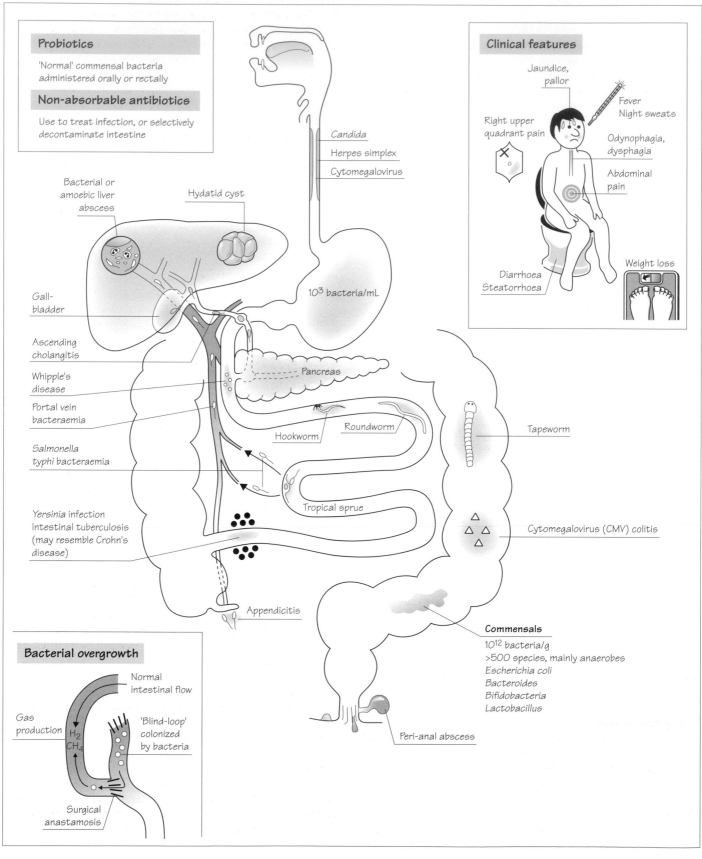

Probiotics

'Normal' commensal bacteria administered orally or rectally

Non-absorbable antibiotics

Use to treat infection, or selectively decontaminate intestine

Bacterial or amoebic liver abscess

Hydatid cyst

Gall-bladder

Ascending cholangitis

Whipple's disease

Portal vein bacteraemia

Salmonella typhi bacteraemia

Yersinia infection
Intestinal tuberculosis (may resemble Crohn's disease)

Candida

Herpes simplex

Cytomegalovirus

10^3 bacteria/mL

Pancreas

Hookworm

Roundworm

Tropical sprue

Tapeworm

Cytomegalovirus (CMV) colitis

Clinical features

Jaundice, pallor

Fever
Night sweats

Right upper quadrant pain

Odynophagia, dysphagia

Abdominal pain

Diarrhoea
Steatorrhoea

Weight loss

Appendicitis

Commensals
10^{12} bacteria/g
>500 species, mainly anaerobes
Escherichia coli
Bacteroides
Bifidobacteria
Lactobacillus

Bacterial overgrowth

Normal intestinal flow

Gas production

H_2
CH_4

'Blind-loop' colonized by bacteria

Surgical anastamosis

Peri-anal abscess

In addition to gastroenteritis and food poisoning, microorganisms cause various other gastrointestinal system-related illness. Furthermore, there is a large resident or commensal population of bacteria, whose role in health and disease remains unknown.

Commensal flora

Bacteria colonize the entire intestinal tract, with the greatest number, 10^{12}/g, in the **large intestine**. They apparently cause no harm and potentially benefit the host, possibly by excluding pathogenic species. There are over **500 different species** and the dominant species and genera are *Escherichia coli*, *Bifidobacteria* and *Lactobacillus*.

E. coli, *Enterococcus*, *Streptococcus*, *Clostridia* and others retain the ability to cause disease, either by acquiring virulence factors, which are usually plasmid or phage DNA-encoding **toxins**, **adhesins**, etc., or by exploiting reduced host defence. *Clostridium difficile*, for example, causes diarrhoea when antibiotic treatment upsets the normal microbial population, allowing it to produce its cytotoxin.

Bacterial overgrowth

The small intestine normally contains very few bacteria because of the constant movement of food and the effect of antimicrobial proteins produced by Paneth cells, for example. Bacteria overgrow, however, when the normal anatomy is disrupted, for example **surgically**, or where diseases like systemic sclerosis cause **dysmotility and stasis**.

The bacteria metabolize nutrients, thus depriving the patient, and produce excess intestinal gas, damage the mucosa and cause **malabsorption**. Symptoms include abdominal pain and flatulence. **Breath tests** can be used to establish the diagnosis. **Antibiotics** and corrective surgery may be necessary.

Worms and parasites

Multicellular worms and parasites commonly infest the intestine, particularly where sanitation is poor. **Hookworms**, **tapeworms** and **roundworms** can remain in the intestine for many years, causing chronic diarrhoea, malabsorption and **anaemia**. Roundworms invade the intestine and migrate through the lungs as part of their life cycle, causing systemic disease. The pork tape-worm, *Taenia solium*, leaves encysted eggs throughout the body, causing **cysticercosis**. Treatment requires **helminthicides** such as albendazole.

Candidiasis

Candida albicans, the only major fungal pathogen of the intestinal tract, is a commensal in most people. Reduced immunity, as in **neutropenia**, **diabetes mellitus**, **steroid use** or acquired immune deficiency syndrome (**AIDS**) allows *Candida* to invade the superficial epithelial layers of the tongue, mouth, pharynx and oesophagus, causing inflammation and pain. Diagnosis is confirmed by detecting fungal hyphae in cytological specimens, or by culture. Topical or systemic **antifungals** such as nystatin or fluconazole are effective therapy.

Whipple's disease

This rare, chronic, intestinal infection caused by *Tropheryma whippelii* typically affects middle-aged Caucasian males, resulting in diarrhoea, malabsorption and fever. Duodenal biopsy shows macrophages containing many bacteria and the treatment is a prolonged course of antibiotics.

Tropical sprue

Chronic diarrhoea and malabsorption, associated with enteric infection, which used to be common in long-term residents of the tropics is now disappearing. **Duodenal biopsy** demonstrates blunt villi and hyperplastic crypts, resembling coeliac disease, and antibiotics are curative.

Systemic infection, abscesses and masses

Intestinal bacteria can migrate into the **portal vein** and form **liver abscesses**, while some enteric organisms, especially streptococci from the mouth and gut, can cause infective **endocarditis**. Therefore, people with valvular heart disease have prophylactic antibiotics before dental and some endoscopic procedures. *Salmonella typhi* causes systemic infection and in immunocompromised patients, less virulent, non-typhi *Salmonella* species can also cause **osteomyelitis**, **brain abscess**, **endocarditis**, etc.

Entamoeba histolytica causes **liver abscess** and abdominal wall masses (**ameoboma**) as well as acute dysentery.

Echinococcus species (**hydatid** worm), acquired from sheep and dogs, invade the intestinal wall, spread systemically and form large, egg-filled cysts in the liver, lungs and other organs.

Liver abscesses typically cause abdominal pain, fever and abnormal blood tests, although they may be asymptomatic. Ultrasound and computerized tomography (CT) scanning are used to make the diagnosis and antibiotics, with or without surgical drainage, are used to treat bacterial and amoebic abscesses. Hydatid disease requires surgical treatment.

Peri-anal abscesses, arising from anaerobic infection of the deep anal glands, are relatively common and are treated by incision and drainage and antibiotics. Recurrent peri-anal sepsis may indicate **anorectal Crohn's** disease.

Inflammatory bowel disease

IBD is not caused by a discrete intestinal infection, although both ulcerative colitis (UC) and Crohn's are triggered by environmental factors that are almost certainly enteric microbes or their products. Antibiotics are generally ineffective in UC, but do improve some forms of Crohn's disease, and administering **probiotics**, which are live commensal bacteria, ameliorates some forms of IBD.

Intestinal infection with *Mycobacterium tuberculosis* and *Yersinia* **species** can strikingly resemble ileocaecal Crohn's disease. Similarly, bacterial and amoebic **dysentery**, cytomegalovirus and herpes simplex virus infection can cause bloody diarrhoea, abdominal pain and intestinal ulceration that can be confused with UC.

Clinical presentation and diagnosis

Chronic intestinal infections can cause abdominal pain, diarrhoea, flatulence, weight loss, malabsorption and/or anaemia.

Stool **culture** can detect **bacterial pathogens** and microscopy can detect **ova**, **cysts and parasites**. Radiological imaging, endoscopy with biopsy and culture, blood culture and serological tests detect deep-seated abscesses and distant infection.

Treatment

The potential role of enteric commensals in health and disease is a reminder that **antibiotics** should be used cautiously. Conversely, live bacteria or **probiotics** may be used therapeutically in certain circumstances.

Selective enteric decontamination, with non-absorbed antibiotics, such as neomycin and norfloxacin, can be used before **intestinal surgery** and in chronic liver disease, to treat **hepatic encephalopathy** and to prevent **spontaneous bacterial peritonitis**. The intestine is not sterilized but the balance of species is altered.

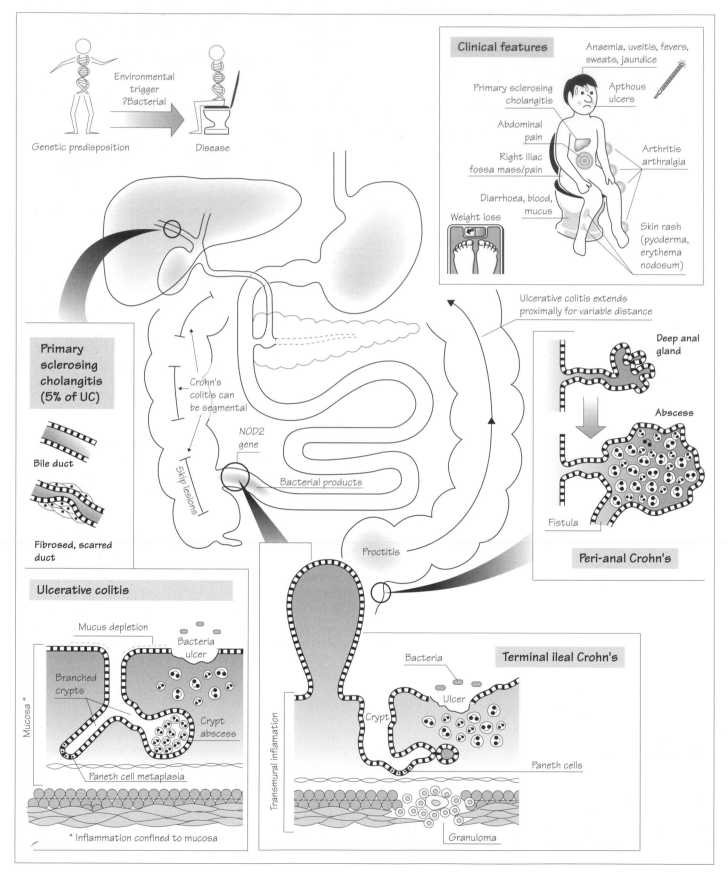

Environmental trigger ?Bacterial

Genetic predisposition → Disease

Clinical features

Anaemia, uveitis, fevers, sweats, jaundice

Primary sclerosing cholangitis

Apthous ulcers

Abdominal pain

Right iliac fossa mass/pain

Arthritis arthralgia

Diarrhoea, blood, mucus

Weight loss

Skin rash (pyoderma, erythema nodosum)

Ulcerative colitis extends proximally for variable distance

Primary sclerosing cholangitis (5% of UC)

Bile duct

Fibrosed, scarred duct

Crohn's colitis can be segmental

Skip lesions

NOD2 gene

Bacterial products

Deep anal gland

Abscess

Fistula

Peri-anal Crohn's

Proctitis

Ulcerative colitis

Mucus depletion

Bacteria ulcer

Branched crypts

Crypt abscess

Mucosa *

Paneth cell metaplasia

* Inflammation confined to mucosa

Transmural inflamation

Terminal ileal Crohn's

Bacteria

Ulcer

Crypt

Paneth cells

Granuloma

Two diseases constitute idiopathic inflammatory bowel disease (**IBD**): **ulcerative colitis** (UC) and **Crohn's** disease (CD). They are distinct but similar, and both are chronic, relapsing and remitting conditions. Together they affect about 150/100 000 of the population in Western countries.

Aetiology

The intestine is constantly in contact with the harsh digestive environment and may be regarded as being in a state of chronic low-grade inflammation. Challenges to the intestine include **pH extremes**, **mechanical trauma**, ingested bacterial and viral **pathogens** and **toxins**, and the microorganisms that comprise the **resident commensal microflora** of the bowel. **Immunological reactivity** may, therefore, develop to components of the diet or the microflora.

The aetiology of IBD remains unknown and it probably results from one or more **environmental triggers** acting against a background of inherited **genetic predisposition**.

Recently, CD of the terminal ileum has been genetically linked to mutations in the *NOD2* gene, which is probably an intracellular receptor for bacterial cell wall components, expressed in monocytes and Paneth cells.

Furthermore, experimentally disrupting the immune system in laboratory animals often leads to intestinal inflammation, which only develops when **enteric bacteria** are present.

Ulcerative colitis and CD may have a number of different primary causes, all resulting in similar clinical and pathological outcomes.

Macroscopic pathology

Ulcerative colitis only affects the large intestine and does not extend to the small intestine. Furthermore, the rectum is almost invariably affected and inflammation extends proximally to a variable extent.

Crohn's disease can affect any part of the intestinal tract, although three patterns predominate: **terminal ileal** inflammation, **colitis** and **anorectal** inflammation. An individual patient could have one, two or three of these areas affected, in any combination. Furthermore, while inflammation in UC is contiguous, extending for a variable distance from the rectum, in CD there may be normal areas interspersed between inflamed segments: '**skip lesions**'.

Microscopic pathology

The mucosa is **ulcerated** and there is an inflammatory reaction in the lamina propria.

In UC, there are reduced numbers of goblet cells (**goblet cell depletion**) and increased numbers of **Paneth cells**. Furthermore, while normal colonic **crypts** are short and straight, in UC they are **distorted** and **branched**. Another typical feature is a collection of neutrophils within the crypt lumen, forming **crypt abscesses**.

Within the lamina propria there are increased numbers of inflammatory cells. The inflammatory reaction in UC does not extend deeper than the **lamina propria**. In contrast, in CD, inflammation typically extends **transmurally** through the wall of the intestine. In addition, there are **granulomas** in CD, consisting of activated lymphocytes and macrophages.

Clinical features

Colitis (UC or Crohn's colitis) causes **diarrhoea**, which usually contains **blood** and pus or mucus. In addition, there may be **abdominal pain** and **malaise** due to the systemic response to inflammation.

In CD, terminal ileitis may cause diarrhoea or constipation, abdominal pain and a palpable **inflammatory mass** in the right iliac fossa. Chronic terminal ileitis may interfere with absorption of **vitamin B_{12}** and **bile salts**, causing **anaemia** and predisposing to gallstones. Inflammation may also cause strictures, resulting in intestinal obstruction.

In CD, because the inflammation extends transmurally, intestinal **fistulae** and deep-seated **abscesses** occur.

The systemic inflammatory response characterized by **fever**, **malaise** and **weight loss** tends to be milder in UC and more pronounced in CD.

Extra-intestinal features of IBD include skin rashes, such as **pyoderma gangrenosum** and **erythema nodosum**, arthralgia and **arthritis** (in up to 15% of patients), and inflammation of the eyes (**iritis** and **uveitis**). **Apthous ulcers** in the mouth are particularly common.

Longstanding UC predisposes to colon cancer and primary sclerosing cholangitis (PSC) occurs in about 5% of patients with UC.

Diagnosis

The mainstay of diagnosing colitis is to perform **sigmoidoscopy** and **colonoscopy**, with mucosal biopsies to histologically confirm the diagnosis. A **barium meal and follow-through** examination visualizes the terminal ileum, demonstrating inflammation, fistulae and strictures. There are no specific blood tests for UC or CD, but **anaemia**, vitamin B_{12} deficiency, and raised inflammatory markers, such as the **C-reactive protein**, are common. In a proportion of UC patients, antineutrophil cytoplasmic antibodies (**ANCA**) are found, while in CD, antibodies to *Saccharomyces cerevisiae* (**ASCA**) may be detected.

Treatment

- **5-Aminosalicylic acid (5ASA, mesalazine)**. This compound has a local anti-inflammatory action, particularly in the colon, and can be administered rectally or orally. Slow release formulations (pentasa or asacol) dissolve in the colon, while conjugated forms of 5ASA (sulphasalazine, olsalazine and balsalazide) are enzymatically released in the colon by bacteria.
- **Corticosteroids**. Steroid treatment is usually effective at inducing remission and is used particularly to treat acute exacerbations. It may be administered parenterally, orally or rectally. Prolonged systemic steroid treatment has many adverse effects, including worsening osteoporosis. **Budesonide** is a synthetic steroid that is rapidly metabolized by the liver, resulting in low systemic levels, and it may be particularly effective for terminal ileal CD.
- **Immunosuppressives**. Drugs such as azathioprine, 6-mercaptopurine and methotrexate are used, particularly when frequent relapses necessitate repeated steroid use. Antibodies to the cytokine tumour necrosis factor α (TNFα) are dramatically effective in a proportion of people with CD.
- **Antibiotics**. Metronidazole may induce remission in some cases of CD but is not effective in UC.
- **Probiotics**. Live bacteria, to restore the normal balance of enteric flora, are used with some success.
- **Surgery**. **Panproctocolectomy** (removal of the colon and rectum) is curative for UC and is used as a last resort for severe disease or where dysplasia develops. CD almost invariably recurs after surgery; therefore the use of surgery is largely limited to, for example, relieving symptomatic strictures or draining abscesses.

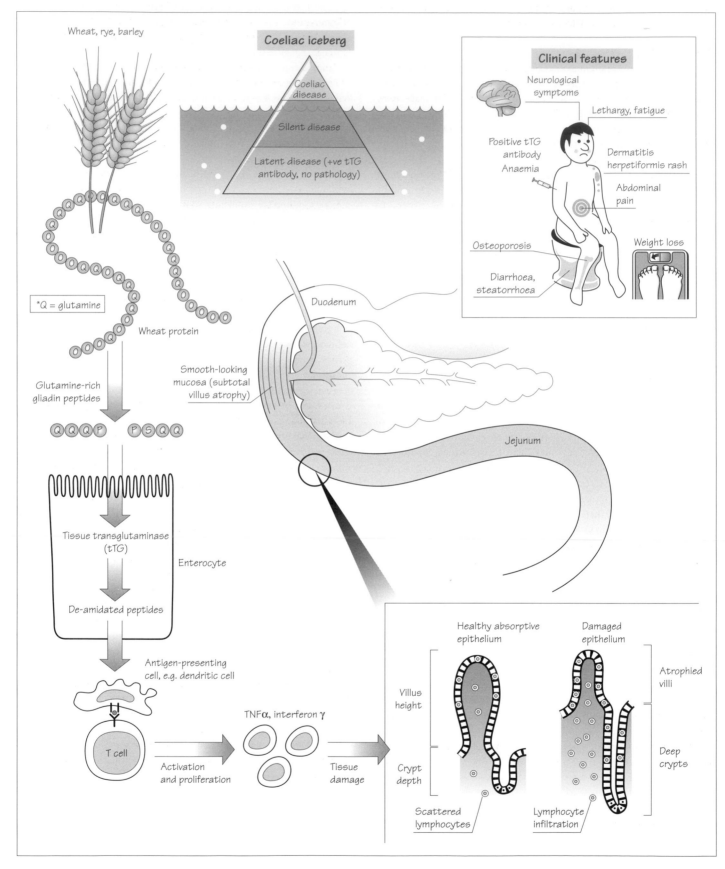

Wheat, rye, barley

Coeliac iceberg

Coeliac disease

Silent disease

Latent disease (+ve tTG antibody, no pathology)

*Q = glutamine

Wheat protein

Glutamine-rich gliadin peptides

Q Q Q P   P S Q Q

Tissue transglutaminase (tTG)

Enterocyte

De-amidated peptides

Antigen-presenting cell, e.g. dendritic cell

T cell

Activation and proliferation

TNFα, interferon γ

Tissue damage

Clinical features

Neurological symptoms

Lethargy, fatigue

Positive tTG antibody
Anaemia

Dermatitis herpetiformis rash

Abdominal pain

Osteoporosis

Weight loss

Diarrhoea, steatorrhoea

Duodenum

Smooth-looking mucosa (subtotal villus atrophy)

Jejunum

Healthy absorptive epithelium

Damaged epithelium

Villus height

Atrophied villi

Crypt depth

Deep crypts

Scattered lymphocytes

Lymphocyte infiltration

Coeliac disease is also known as **gluten enteropathy** because it is caused by immune reactivity triggered by glutamine- and proline-rich gluten proteins, found mainly in **wheat**, **rye**, **barley** and **oats**. The illness may become apparent at any age, from infancy to old age, may remain asymptomatic, and may be detected incidentally.

Aetiology and pathogenesis

The healthy small intestinal epithelium is maintained by constant cell turnover, and the balance between normal shedding of old epithelial cells at the tips of villi and the formation of new cells from **stem cells** in the crypts maintains a **2 : 1 ratio** between villus height and crypt depth. The **lamina propria** contains a small number of lymphocytes, macrophages, fibroblasts, capillary endothelial cells and other cells. The epithelium itself contains a population of resident **intraepithelial lymphocytes** that maintain **surveillance** against potential pathogens.

In **genetically susceptible** individuals, immunological reaction to gluten-derived **gliadin** peptides develops upon dietary exposure. The exact genes causing coeliac disease have not been identified but certain major histocompatibility complex (**MHC**) **class II** gene alleles are strongly associated with the condition. Early dietary exposure to gluten, particularly after **weaning** from milk, may increase the risk of developing the disease.

The ubiquitous cellular enzyme **tissue transglutaminase (tTG)**, which normally cross-links glutamine residues with lysine in connective tissue proteins, plays an essential role in the pathogenesis, by converting glutamine residues in native gliadin peptides to glutamate, creating more immunogenic peptides. However no disease-associated polymorphisms in the *tTG* gene have been identified.

Lymphocytes react with the modified gliadin peptides on the surface of **antigen-presenting cells** and proliferate, increasing the number of intraepithelial and lamina propria lymphocytes. Activated lymphocytes secrete inflammatory mediators, including the **cytokines**, γ-interferon and tumour necrosis factor α (**TNFα**), **recruiting** and **activating** more inflammatory cells, altering the **proliferative rate** of intestinal epithelial **stem cells**, and increasing the rate of programmed cell death (**apoptosis**) in mature enterocytes. This creates an oedematous, swollen intestinal mucosa, with short, thick, blunt villi and deeper than normal crypts (**subtotal villus atrophy**), and the reduced epithelial surface area and compromised epithelial digestive and absorptive capacity leads to **malabsorption**.

The concentration of dietary gluten is highest proximally in the intestine and therefore coeliac disease affects the duodenum and proximal jejunum most severely.

Clinical features

Coeliac disease can become apparent at **any age**, although most cases are diagnosed in early childhood or in middle age. Coeliac disease may remain clinically silent and people with circulating antibodies to tTG, but no overt pathology, may be considered to have latent disease.

Malabsorption causes **diarrhoea** and **weight loss**. Inability to absorb fats results in **steatorrhoea**, with bulky, pale, foul-smelling stools that float in water, because of their high fat content. **Anaemia**, caused by iron deficiency is frequent. Malabsorption of calcium and vitamin D increases the risk of developing **osteoporosis**.

Nutrients that are mainly absorbed in the proximal small intestine, such as **iron** and **calcium**, are most affected by coeliac disease, while nutrients predominantly absorbed in the jejunum and ileum, such as **folic acid**, **vitamin C** and **vitamin B$_{12}$**, are affected only in more advanced disease.

Patients may complain of **abdominal pain** and **tiredness** and, for unknown reasons, **neurological complaints**, ranging from mild peripheral neuropathy to more severe central nervous system disturbance, occur in up to 10% of patients.

A small number of people develop a blistering rash called **dermatitis herpetiformis**, associated with antibodies to tTG reacting with a form of this enzyme in dermal cells.

Possibly as the result of chronic inflammation, people with uncontrolled coeliac disease are at increased risk of developing intestinal **neoplasms**, particularly intestinal **lymphoma**. This risk is substantially reduced by strict adherence to a gliadin-free diet (see Chapter 38).

All these signs and symptoms disappear when gliadin is omitted from the diet and reappear if it is reintroduced.

Diagnosis

Unexplained anaemia and vague abdominal and neurological symptoms should prompt the physician to check for coeliac disease, as it is often missed and is particularly common in some populations, such as people originating from western Ireland. Conversely, it remains rare among Africans.

Circulating **antibodies** to tTG offer an excellent serological marker of coeliac disease, with sensitivity and specificity approaching 100%. The test was first described as detecting an unknown antigen in the lining of oesophageal smooth muscle (endomysium), hence the term **anti-endomysial antibody**. This test replaces the **antigliadin** anti-body test that has lower sensitivity and specificity. Serological tests rely on detecting immunoglobulin A (**IgA**) antibodies and are unreliable in the 1 : 500 individuals with selective IgA deficiency (see Chapter 18).

Upper gastrointestinal **endoscopy** and duodenal **mucosal biopsy**, to confirm **subtotal villus atrophy** and lymphocytic infiltration, is performed before treatment, after initiating a gliadin-free diet, and again after reintroduction of a gliadin challenge diet, and is the gold standard of diagnosis. With the advent of reliable serological testing, it is now used less frequently.

Rare forms of small intestinal disease, such as Whipple's disease, Crohn's disease of the small intestine and **tropical sprue** may mimic coeliac disease and here a duodenal or jejunal biopsy may be particularly helpful in the diagnosis.

Treatment

The mainstay of treatment is for patients to follow a **gluten-free diet**. Wheat, rye and barley proteins are present in many ready-made meals and snacks, so the help of a professional dietician and a patients' association, such as the **Coeliac Society** in the UK, should be enlisted to maintain vigilance. In severe, uncontrolled coeliac disease, acute intestinal inflammation can be treated with corticosteroids, but this is hazardous and rarely indicated.

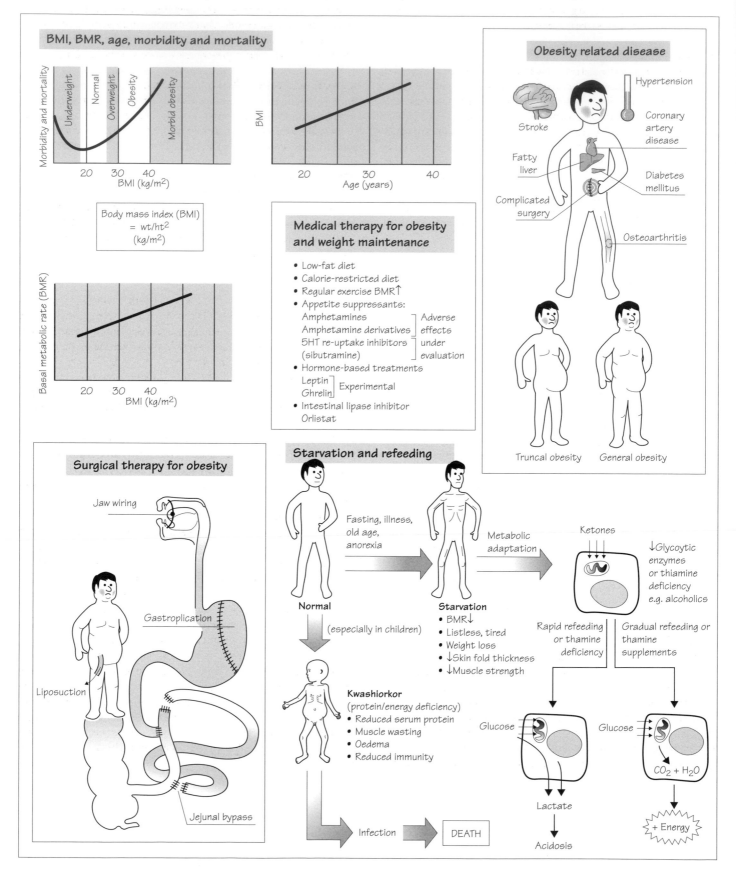

BMI, BMR, age, morbidity and mortality

Body mass index (BMI)
= wt/ht^2
(kg/m^2)

Obesity related disease

Stroke
Hypertension
Coronary artery disease
Fatty liver
Diabetes mellitus
Complicated surgery
Osteoarthritis

Truncal obesity   General obesity

Medical therapy for obesity and weight maintenance

- Low-fat diet
- Calorie-restricted diet
- Regular exercise BMR↑
- Appetite suppressants:
  Amphetamines ⎤
  Amphetamine derivatives ⎥ Adverse effects
  5HT re-uptake inhibitors ⎥ under evaluation
  (sibutramine) ⎦
- Hormone-based treatments
  Leptin ⎤ Experimental
  Ghrelin ⎦
- Intestinal lipase inhibitor Orlistat

Surgical therapy for obesity

Jaw wiring
Gastroplication
Liposuction
Jejunal bypass

Starvation and refeeding

Fasting, illness, old age, anorexia

Normal

Metabolic adaptation

Starvation
- BMR↓
- Listless, tired
- Weight loss
- ↓Skin fold thickness
- ↓Muscle strength

Ketones

↓Glycoytic enzymes or thiamine deficiency e.g. alcoholics

Rapid refeeding or thamine deficiency

Gradual refeeding or thamine supplements

(especially in children)

Kwashiorkor
(protein/energy deficiency)
- Reduced serum protein
- Muscle wasting
- Oedema
- Reduced immunity

Glucose

Glucose

$CO_2 + H_2O$

Infection → DEATH

Lactate

Acidosis

+ Energy

Obesity

Obesity is arguably the most prevalent health problem in the Western world and its incidence is increasing worldwide. Body weight is tightly regulated so that strategies to gain or lose weight must overcome strong homeostatic mechanisms (see Chapter 22).

Measuring obesity

Obesity implies an abnormal ratio of adipose tissue to lean mass (mainly bone and muscle). The body mass index (BMI) (weight in kg/(height in m)^2) is a practical guide to healthy body weight. The normal BMI is between 18 and 25; over 25 is overweight, over 30 is obese and over 40 is morbidly obese. Skin-fold thickness also measures body fat stores, as does total body impedance to a low frequency electrical current, and total body density, which can be determined in research settings.

Obesity is associated with excessive rates of illness, particularly **hypertension**, **diabetes** mellitus, **stroke**, vascular **thrombosis** and **heart disease**. A simple measure of overweight that correlates with the risk of cardiovascular disease is the **waist : hip ratio**, with the normal ratio being less than one.

Treating obesity

Body weight tends to increase with age, and preventing obesity is as important as reducing weight.

- **Diet**. Restricting **calorie intake** reduces body weight. Initial weight loss tends to be followed by **rebound** weight gain after a few months. Some diets restrict **fluid intake** and dehydration causes rapid but spurious weight loss. To **maintain weight** control, diets must be **sustainable** and nutritionally adequate and not lack essential vitamins, minerals or macronutrients. **Very low calorie diets**, carry the risk of undernutrition and should be supervised by a physician, while **low calorie diets**, for example, those advocated by WeightWatchers™, are safer.

Large **portions** and a preponderance of **calorie-dense foods**, that is, fats, tend to increase calorie intake. Ideally the proportion of calories consumed as fat should be between 20 and 30% of the total.

- **Exercise**. Regular exercise helps to limit body weight, partly by **consuming calories** to provide energy to muscle and also by **suppressing appetite** and raising the **basal metabolic rate** (BMR) (see Chapter 22).
- **Pharmacotherapy**. The medical consequences of obesity are being increasingly recognized and effective treatments actively sought, partly stimulated by the discovery of **leptin** and other endogenous appetite-suppressants, and the results of research into neuro-endocrine control of body weight.

The most effective appetite suppressants were the **amphetamine** derivatives dexfenfluramine and phenteramine, which unfortunately caused major cardiac side-effects and were withdrawn from use. **Sibutramine** is another effective appetite suppressant acting through **serotoninergic** pathways. Orlistat is a specific **pancreatic lipase inhibitor** that causes fat malabsorption and weight loss. Side-effects, such as oily stool and fat-soluble vitamin deficiencies, limit its use.

- Occasionally, obesity is caused by **endocrine dysfunction**, such as hypothyroidism, and treating the underlying condition is effective.
- **Surgery**. Surgical removal of fat, for example, by liposuction and gastrointestinal surgery to limit food intake and absorption are the main options. Cosmetic surgery has only short-term benefits and risks scarring and infection. Gastrointestinal surgery is reserved for treating morbid obesity. **Jejuno-ileal bypass** is no longer performed, because it caused severe liver disease (**steatohepatitis**). **Jaw-wiring**, which limits food intake, and **gastroplication**, whereby a portion of the stomach is stitched or enclosed with a rubber band, reducing the size of the gastric reservoir, are the most frequent operations for obesity (see Chapter 48).

Starvation, malnutrition and anorexia

Malnutrition has many causes, of which economic deprivation is the commonest. However, even in wealthy societies, ill health, gastrointestinal diseases, such as oesophageal cancer, and anorexia nervosa, as well as voluntary fasting, can all cause malnutrition and starvation.

Measuring malnutrition

The **BMI** is abnormally low and other measures, such as **skin-fold thickness** and muscle strength and mass, are low. **Listlessness** and **lethargy** occur and with severe starvation, **multiple organ failure** may occur. In women, **menstruation** ceases. There may also be signs of specific vitamin and mineral deficiencies.

Effects of malnutrition

Malnutrition causes widespread abnormalities, including changes in the **gastrointestinal tract**. Villi are shorter, less digestive enzymes are synthesized and the intestinal barrier to the entry of pathogens is reduced. This **atrophy** occurs whenever the intestine is not used, so patients who are fed **parenterally** are also at risk. Malnourished children have stunted growth and, due to mucosal atrophy and a general reduction in immune competence, are particularly susceptible to infections, such as **gastroenteritis**, which aggravates the malnutrition and may be fatal.

Metabolic adaptation, which reduces dependence on glucose and lowers the BMR, allows the organism to survive for longer at a lower energy intake. An important consequence is that rapid refeeding after a period of starvation can induce serious metabolic abnormalities (**refeeding syndrome**).

Kwashiorkor, or protein-energy malnutrition, occurs when protein deficiency is greater than overall calorie deficiency. Tissue and blood proteins are inadequately renewed, causing skin, hair and serum protein abnormalities and, characteristically, peripheral **oedema**. **Marasmus**, in contrast, is global malnutrition, without oedema.

Specific micronutrient deficiencies also occur in malnutrition and, paradoxically, global malnutrition may mask specific vitamin deficiencies. For example, malnourished alcohol-dependent people, who neglect nutrition in favour of alcohol, may be **thiamine** (vitamin B$_1$) deficient. The deficiency may not be clinically apparent while they consume a diet lacking carbohydrates. However, if they are admitted to hospital and given intravenous glucose or a good meal, acute thiamine deficiency occurs, because thiamine is an essential cofactor for the pyruvate dehydrogenase enzyme, which metabolizes glucose in cells. Acute thiamine deficiency is a medical emergency and can cause permanent neurological damage (**Wernicke's encephalopathy**) if thiamine is not administered immediately.

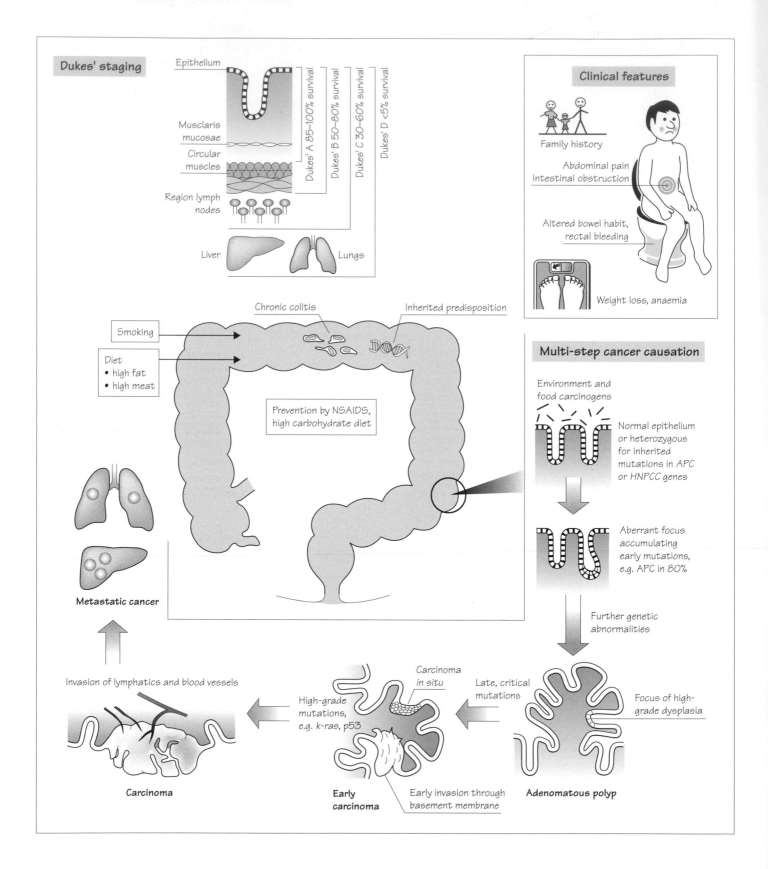

Dukes' staging

Epithelium

Musclaris mucosae

Circular muscles

Region lymph nodes

Dukes' A 85–100% survival
Dukes' B 50–80% survival
Dukes' C 30–60% survival
Dukes' D <5% survival

Liver — Lungs

Clinical features

Family history

Abdominal pain
Intestinal obstruction

Altered bowel habit, rectal bleeding

Weight loss, anaemia

Chronic colitis — Inherited predisposition

Smoking

Diet
• high fat
• high meat

Prevention by NSAIDS, high carbohydrate diet

Multi-step cancer causation

Environment and food carcinogens

Normal epithelium or heterozygous for inherited mutations in APC or HNPCC genes

Aberrant focus accumulating early mutations, e.g. APC in 80%

Further genetic abnormalities

Metastatic cancer

Invasion of lymphatics and blood vessels

Carcinoma in situ

High-grade mutations, e.g. k-ras, p53

Late, critical mutations

Focus of high-grade dysplasia

Carcinoma

Early carcinoma

Early invasion through basement membrane

Adenomatous polyp

Gastrointestinal cancers impose a major health burden: colon and rectal cancer (**colorectal cancer**, **CRC**) is the second commonest cause of cancer-related death in the Western world, while gastric, oesophageal, pancreatic and liver cancer are also relatively frequent.

Pathology

The development of colorectal cancer follows a characteristic pattern in most cases, with the earliest lesion being a microscopic focus of **aberrant epithelial cells**. With time these form a small **dysplastic polyp**, which enlarges, comprising epithelial cells with increasing numbers of mutations in cancer-related genes and a progressively dysplastic phenotype.

Some cells may become malignant, forming a focus of **carcinoma in situ**, which is confined to the epithelium of the polyp. These malignant cells may penetrate the basement membrane and invade first the intestinal wall and then **lymphatics** via which they are carried to regional lymph nodes. Finally they may invade **blood vessels** and so **metastasize** to distant organs such as the liver and lungs.

The **Dukes staging** is used to determine prognosis and optimal treatment (see figure).

Aetiology and pathogenesis

Environmental factors including **diet** influence the incidence of CRC. Western diets that are high in **fat** and **red meat** and low in **fibre** predispose to CRC, while vegetables, vitamins, trace elements, such as selenium, and non-steroidal anti-inflammatory drugs (NSAIDs), such as sulindac, seem to be protective. **Smoking** tobacco also increases the risk of CRC. High-fat diets induce the production of **carcinogens**, while reduced dietary fibre causes **constipation** so that the carcinogens remain in contact with the epithelium for longer.

Chronic intestinal inflammation, as in ulcerative colitis, also increases the risk, possibly by increasing epithelial cell turnover, and thus increasing the chance of genetic mutations.

There is a strong **genetic** element and the risk of CRC is increased in people who have one or more affected first-degree relatives. The study of familial forms of CRC, particularly autosomal dominant **familial adenomatous polyposis** (FAP) and **hereditary non-polyposis colon cancer** (HNPCC), have helped to elucidate the molecular pathogenesis of CRC, based on the '**two-hit**' **and multiple gene theory** of how tumour suppressor genes function.

Colonic epithelial cells undergo **progressive change** from normal, through increasing dysplasia, to carcinoma. These cellular changes are caused by genetic changes; some of which may be inherited and others acquired through the effect of carcinogens. Mutation of a single allele is usually insufficient to alter cellular function, so, for each gene, both alleles must be mutated.

In genetic CRC syndromes, one mutant allele is inherited, so only a single second mutation in that gene is required. To produce cancer, numerous genes must be mutated; therefore, it takes many years to accumulate sufficient mutations. For example, FAP is caused by mutations in the **adenomatous polyposis coli** (**APC**) gene, which is frequently mutated even in sporadic, non-familial CRC. Patients with FAP develop many hundreds of polyps and then cancer in their early 20s in almost all cases. This occurs because each colonocyte already carries one mutated *APC* gene, so that environmental carcinogens only have to mutate and inactivate the single remaining copy to produce a polyp, which can then go on to develop into a cancer.

HNPCC does not involve a polyp-forming stage and is associated with mutations in the genes responsible for ensuring that mistakes in copying DNA during mitosis are repaired (**mismatch repair genes**). Patients lose the ability to correct genetic mistakes and thus accumulate mutations in neoplasia-inducing genes, including ACP, **p53** and *k-ras*.

Clinical features

Except in familial syndromes, CRC is rare before the age of **50 years** and it increases in incidence thereafter. Early cancers and adenomas in the colon may remain entirely **asymptomatic**. Larger adenomas and cancers may bleed microscopically over time, causing **anaemia**. Larger tumours may cause overt **rectal bleeding** and **altered bowel habit** (constipation and/or diarrhoea). Intestinal obstruction, abdominal pain and weight loss occur when the disease is further advanced.

Diagnosis

Barium enema and **colonoscopy** are the main diagnostic tests. **Histology** of colonic polyp biopsies can demonstrate dysplasia and neoplasia (see Chapters 44 & 45).

Stool examination may demonstrate occult bleeding. **Faecal occult blood** testing is based on the guiaic chemical reaction with haem, and false positives may be caused by dietary haem, for example, from meat (see Chapter 43).

Blood tests may show iron deficiency or **anaemia**. Increased circulating levels of an embryonic protein, carcino-embryonic antigen (**CEA**), are associated with CRC and can be used to monitor tumour recurrence after surgery and chemotherapy.

Removal of adenomatous polyps before they become malignant dramatically reduces the risk of developing CRC. Therefore, because CRC is so common, some authorities advocate population **screening**, using barium enema, colonoscopy or faecal occult blood testing for people over the age of 50 years.

In FAP, the **panproctocolectomy** (surgical removal of the whole colon and rectum) in early adulthood prevents CRC.

Treatment

- **Surgery**: simple adenomas may be removed during colonoscopy by snaring and excision (**polypectomy**), while CRC has to be removed surgically together with a margin of normal tissue to ensure total resection. If CRC is detected early, particularly if it has not extended beyond the intestinal wall, the operation may be curative. Metastatic CRC cannot be cured, although surgery may palliate symptoms, such as bleeding, obstruction and pain.
- **Chemotherapy and radiotherapy**: adjuvant chemotherapy may increase survival after surgery and radiotherapy may be used to reduce tumour bulk.
- **Prevention**: a diet that is low in fat and red meat and high in carbohydrate and fibre is recommended, and the use of NSAIDs is being investigated.

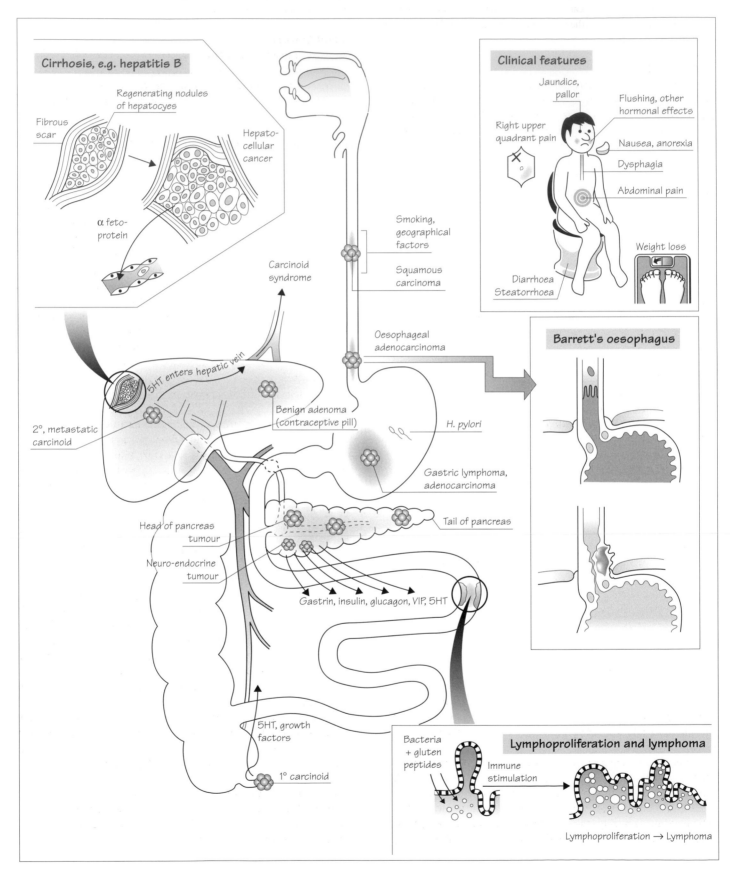

Cirrhosis, e.g. hepatitis B

Regenerating nodules of hepatocyes

Fibrous scar

Hepato-cellular cancer

α feto-protein

Clinical features

Jaundice, pallor

Flushing, other hormonal effects

Right upper quadrant pain

Nausea, anorexia

Dysphagia

Abdominal pain

Weight loss

Diarrhoea
Steatorrhoea

Carcinoid syndrome

5HT enters hepatic vein

Smoking, geographical factors

Squamous carcinoma

Oesophageal adenocarcinoma

Barrett's oesophagus

2°, metastatic carcinoid

Benign adenoma (contraceptive pill)

H. pylori

Gastric lymphoma, adenocarcinoma

Head of pancreas tumour

Neuro-endocrine tumour

Tail of pancreas

Gastrin, insulin, glucagon, VIP, 5HT

5HT, growth factors

1° carcinoid

Lymphoproliferation and lymphoma

Bacteria + gluten peptides

Immune stimulation

Lymphoproliferation → Lymphoma

Tumours of the colon, oesophagus, stomach, pancreas and liver are common worldwide. Colon cancer is the most common (see Chapter 37). There is marked **geographical** and **racial variation** in the incidence of gastric, oesophageal, pancreatic and liver cancer. In cirrhosis, primary liver cancer is common and the liver is also a frequent site for **metastasis** from many other cancers.

Gastric cancer

Gastric cancer is particularly prevalent in Japan, but the **incidence is decreasing** worldwide. Environmental factors, such as **smoked foods**, play a role and **chronic gastritis**, caused by **autoimmune** disease, or more commonly by *Helicobacter pylori* infection, predisposes to both **adenocarcinoma** and gastric **lymphoma** (see Chapter 31).

Symptoms include abdominal pain, dyspepsia, anaemia and occult or overt intestinal bleeding. Advanced cancer may cause a palpable mass in the epigastrium and lymphatic spread may create a palpable lymph node in the neck – '**Virchow's node**'.

Endoscopy may reveal a **gastric ulcer**. All gastric ulcers should be biopsied and a second endoscopy performed after 2 months of treatment to assess healing: non-healing gastric ulcers may be malignant.

Oesophageal cancer

Squamous cell carcinoma of the oesophagus is the commonest form and is particularly prevalent in parts of **southern Africa**. In the Western world, however, the incidence of oesophageal **adenocarcinoma** is increasing.

Squamous cell carcinoma is related to smoking and drinking alcohol, while chronic gastro-oesophageal reflux and **Barrett's oesophagus** predispose to adenocarcinoma. **Chronic reflux** can cause metaplasia of the oesophageal epithelium, from stratified squamous to simple columnar, intestinal-type epithelium. This change is termed Barrett's oesophagus, which carries a risk of dysplasia and subsequent malignant transformation (see Chapters 4 & 30).

Dysphagia (food sticking) and **odynophagia** (pain on swallowing) signify oesophageal disease and may be accompanied by **weight loss**. Malignant tracheo-oesophageal fistulae may cause recurrent aspiration pneumonia. **Barium swallow**, **endoscopy**, biopsy and brush cytology confirm the diagnosis.

Very early disease may be cured by **oesophagectomy** but usually the cancer is non-resectable and patients receive **palliative treatment** by dilatation of strictures, placement of mechanical stents or laser treatment to reduce tumour bulk.

Some authorities advocate regular **endoscopic surveillance** to detect dysplasia in Barrett's oesophagus so adenocarcinoma can be detected and treated early.

Gastrointestinal lymphoma

Gastric and intestinal lymphomas are rare and are usually caused by chronic inflammation and activation of the local immune system, as with *H. pylori* infection, **coeliac disease** and immunoproliferative small intestinal disease (**IPSID**), which occurs with chronic intestinal infection (see Chapters 18, 31 & 35).

Symptoms include **weight loss**, **diarrhoea**, **malabsorption** and abdominal pain. Diagnosis is hampered by the difficulty in reaching parts of the small intestine by endoscopy (see Chapter 44). Barium meal and follow-through examination, computerized tomography (CT), magnetic resonance imaging (MRI) scanning and exploratory laparotomy with intestinal biopsy are often used to make the diagnosis (see Chapter 45).

Eradicating *H. pylori* infection, or prolonged antibiotic treatment of IPSID, may cure early cases. In coeliac disease, strict adherence to a gluten-free diet removes the antigenic stimulus to lymphocytes and reduces the risk of lymphoma.

Pancreatic cancer

Pancreatic **adenocarcinomas** may present with abdominal pain or, when they occur in the head of the pancreas, may obstruct the common bile duct, causing **jaundice**. Very early cancers may be treated by wide excision of the pancreas, duodenum and related structures (**Whipple's operation**).

Neuro-endocrine tumours and carcinoids

Tumours arising from entero-endocrine tissue may be benign or malignant, and may occur sporadically or as part of inherited multiple endocrine neoplasia (**MEN**) syndromes. They may be asymptomatic for many years, or may produce symptoms by virtue of **aberrant hormone secretion**, even while the tumour itself is extremely small and physically inapparent; for example, tumours of G-cell origin produce gastrin, resulting in excess stomach acid production and peptic ulceration (**Zollinger–Ellison** syndrome). Other tumours may produce insulin, glucagon or vasoactive intestinal peptide (VIP), causing diarrhoea and hypokalaemia (**Verner–Morrison** syndrome) (see Chapter 16).

Carcinoids are typically slow-growing tumours that produce an excess of serotonin (5-hydroxytryptamine, **5HT**) and peptide growth factors. They usually remain asymptomatic, as the liver rapidly metabolizes 5HT. However, when carcinoids metastasize to the liver, 5HT is released directly into the systemic circulation, causing symptoms such as **flushing** and **diarrhoea**, which constitute the **carcinoid syndrome**.

Hormonal effects are often the first sign of neuro-endocrine tumours. Anatomical localization can be difficult and relies on CT and MRI imaging and radionuclide-based scans to localize tumour cells expressing surface somatostatin receptors, which are present on most neuro-endocrine tumours (**octreotide scan**). Excess urinary excretion of 5-hydroxy-indole acetic acid (**5-HIAA**), a metabolite of 5HT, can be used to diagnose carcinoid syndrome.

Octreotide or somatostatin injections may alleviate symptoms by suppressing hormone secretion, and surgery is potentially curative.

Liver cancer and masses

Primary liver cancer (**hepatoma**) is rare, except in chronic liver disease and **cirrhosis**, particularly when the liver disease is caused by hepatitis B virus infection. People with primary sclerosing cholangitis (**PSC**) are particularly prone to develop cancer of the biliary epithelium, **cholangiocarcinoma**. Non-malignant **hepatic adenoma** is associated with the use of the **oral contraceptive pill**. The most commonly occurring cancers in the liver are **metastatic deposits** from cancer of the stomach, colon, pancreas and breast.

Typical symptoms include right upper quadrant **pain** and, if the tumour obstructs bile flow, **jaundice**. Serum levels of liver **enzymes** and bilirubin may be raised. In hepatoma, elevated circulating levels of the embryonic protein, **α-fetoprotein** (AFP) may be detected.

Ultrasound, CT and MRI scans and a liver biopsy may be needed to confirm the diagnosis and to distinguish cancer from benign cysts, haemangiomas, abscesses and benign tumours (see Chapters 33 & 45). Treatment remains unsatisfactory.

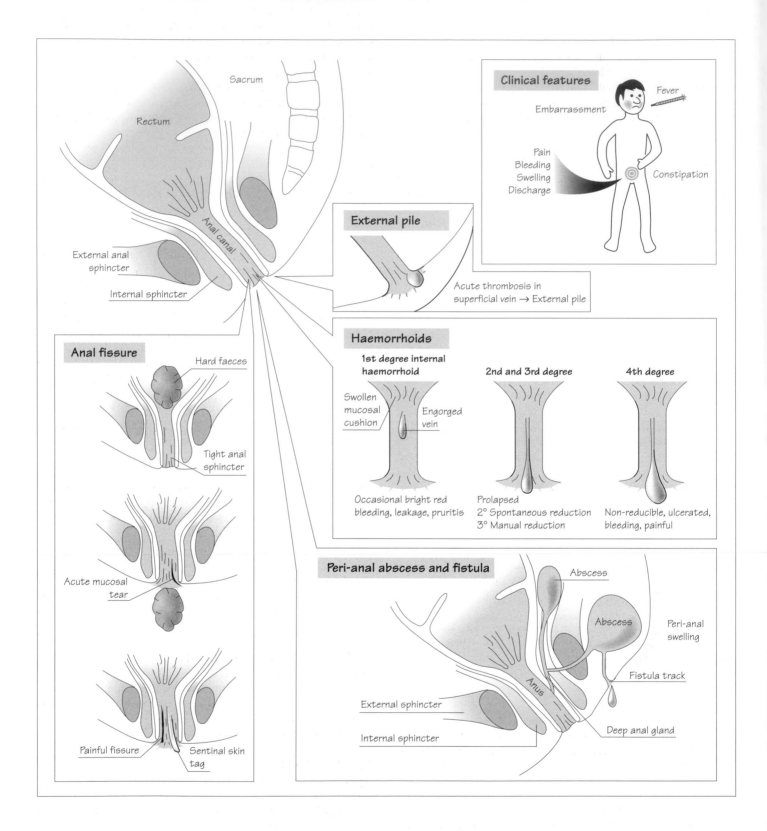

Sacrum

Rectum

Anal canal

External anal sphincter

Internal sphincter

Clinical features

Fever

Embarrassment

Pain
Bleeding
Swelling
Discharge

Constipation

External pile

Acute thrombosis in superficial vein → External pile

Anal fissure

Hard faeces

Tight anal sphincter

Acute mucosal tear

Painful fissure

Sentinal skin tag

Haemorrhoids

1st degree internal haemorrhoid

Swollen mucosal cushion

Engorged vein

Occasional bright red bleeding, leakage, pruritis

2nd and 3rd degree

Prolapsed
2° Spontaneous reduction
3° Manual reduction

4th degree

Non-reducible, ulcerated, bleeding, painful

Peri-anal abscess and fistula

Abscess

Abscess

Peri-anal swelling

Fistula track

Anus

External sphincter

Internal sphincter

Deep anal gland

The peri-anal region is a frequent source of pain, discomfort and distress. Fortunately, many conditions affecting this region are benign and treatable.

Haemorrhoids

Heamorrhoids are commonly known as piles. They may cause rectal **pain** and **bleeding** and may interfere with defecation.

External piles are actually dilated superficial veins in the peri-anal skin, which become thrombosed and exquisitely painful. Occasionally, the thrombosed pile may bleed. When they heal, an external skin tag may remain.

Internal haemorrhoids arise from superficial veins in the mucosa of the **lower rectum**, which become engorged through chronically raised intra-abdominal pressure and **straining** during defecation. The veins are supported by cushions of soft connective tissue, which hypertrophy and contribute to the swelling (see Chapter 14). Chronic straining is the commonest cause of haemorrhoidal vein enlargement and contributing factors include pregnancy, obesity and weight lifting.

First-degree internal haemorrhoids comprise hypertrophied cushions, with enlarged veins that may bleed but do not protrude out of the rectum into the anus.

Second-degree haemorrhoids **prolapse** through the anus, but **reduce spontaneously**.

Third-degree haemorrhoids require **manual reduction** of the prolapse and **fourth-degree haemorrhoids** cannot be reduced manually.

Internal haemorrhoids generally do not cause pain unless they prolapse and ulcerate. They may cause a sense of rectal fullness, discomfort and incomplete evacuation (**tenesmus**). The most common symptoms include **bleeding**, typically at the end of defecation, and the effects of prolapse, which include chronic **leakage** of mucus and subsequent peri-anal itching (**pruritis ani**) and excoriation.

The diagnosis is confirmed by careful examination of the peri-anal region and anal canal using a **proctoscope**. Barium enema and colonoscopy may be needed to exclude other causes of rectal bleeding.

Medical treatment includes altering **diet** to avoid constipation, using **stool softeners** and changing behaviour to avoid straining during defecation.

Surgically, haemorrhoids can be treated by elastic band **ligation**, **sclerotherapy** or **excision**. External piles do not usually require treatment, apart from incision and evacuation of an acutely painful thrombus.

Anal fissure

A split in the skin of the anal canal causes acute **tearing pain**, particularly on defecation. There may also be some **bleeding**. The cause is constipation and hard stool.

On examination, there is a linear tear in the skin. Ninety percent of tears are posterior and 10% anterior. There may be a skin tag, called a **sentinel pile**, at the edge of a chronic tear.

Stool softeners and alleviating constipation are the main treatments and, in the acute state, local application of **glyceryl trinitrate** ointment, which relaxes the anal sphincter, may allow the fissure to heal. In chronic cases, surgical division of the internal anal sphincter (**sphincterotomy**) may be performed.

Anorectal abscess and fistula

The deep anal glands, which secrete mucus into the anal canal, extend between the internal and external sphincters and may become **obstructed** and **infected**. This causes deep-seated peri-anal abscesses that manifest with anal **pain**, **fever** and usually a palpable **peri-anal mass**. When the abscess ruptures onto the surface, a tract or **fistula** may persist and can become chronically infected, **discharging** mucus and pus. Anorectal fistulae may also occur after surgical incision and drainage of abscesses.

Abscesses and fistulae may be deeper than clinically apparent and computerized tomography (**CT**) and magnetic resonance imaging (**MRI**) **scanning** of the pelvis may be helpful before surgical treatment. Surgical **incision and drainage** are usually required and broad-spectrum **antibiotics**, including metronidazole to treat anaerobic infection, are used.

Chronic and recurrent anorectal sepsis may be caused by **anorectal Crohn's disease**, in which case additional anti-inflammatory treatment is also required (see Chapter 34).

Proctitis

Superficial inflammation of the rectal mucosa, causing **bleeding, diarrhoea**, **urgency** of defecation and mucus discharge, may be caused by ulcerative colitis or Crohn's disease. In many cases, inflammation remains confined to the rectum and never extends proximally. Rectal steroids and 5-aminosalicylic acid (5ASA, mesalazine) are usually effective and long-term treatment with oral 5ASA may be initiated.

Radiation proctitis. Pelvic irradiation, for example, to treat cervical cancer in women, or prostrate cancer in men, may cause chronic vascular damage and mucosal fibrosis, with the formation of friable, abnormal blood vessels that bleed spontaneously. The symptoms of diarrhoea, rectal bleeding and discharge may develop years after the initial radiotherapy.

Pruritis ani

Poor perineal hygeine may cause irritation of the peri-anal skin and, conversely, overzealous cleaning with soaps may dry the skin, also causing irritation. Infestation with pinworms (*Enterobius vermicularis*), which crawl onto the peri-anal skin, may also cause pruritis, as might chronic mucus discharge caused by haemorrhoids.

Proctalgia fugax

Proctalgia fugax is a stabbing pain in the rectum, often after defecation, and usually has no discernable organic cause and is hard to treat (see Chapter 29).

Anal warts and sexually transmitted infections

Infection with human papillomavirus may cause peri-anal warts that are treated in the same way as genital warts. Syphilis may also cause wart-like papules, as well as peri-anal ulcers. Other sexually transmitted diseases, such as herpes simplex virus infection and gonorrhoea, may cause peri-anal inflammation and ulceration.

Peri-anal tumours

Squamous cell carcinoma is the most common anal tumour and may be associated with infection by human papillomavirus 16 and 18. Chronic hypertrophic ulcers with rolled edges are the typical manifestation and they may cause bleeding, itching and pain.

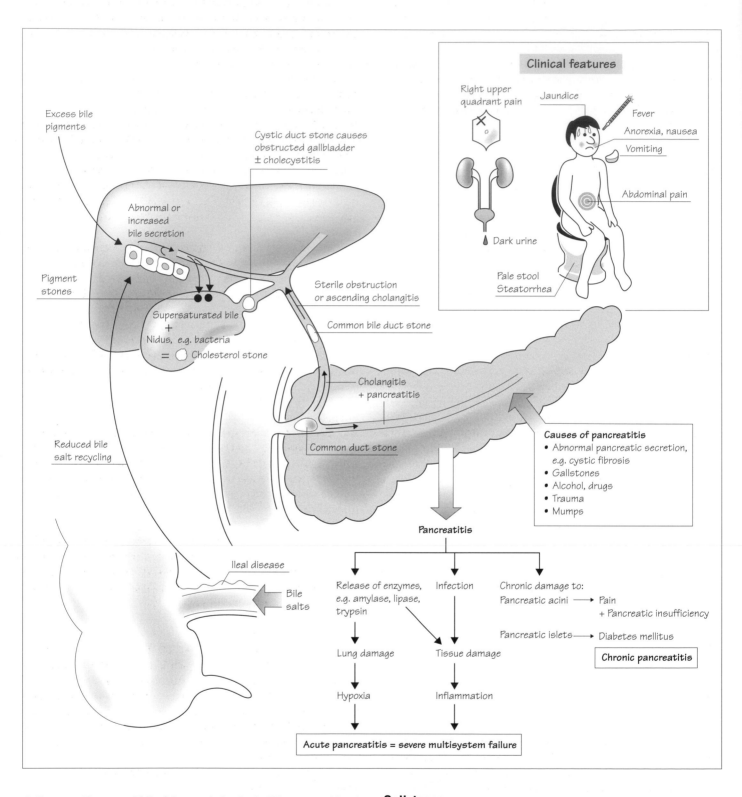

Clinical features

Right upper quadrant pain

Jaundice

Fever

Anorexia, nausea

Vomiting

Abdominal pain

Dark urine

Pale stool
Steatorrhea

Excess bile pigments

Cystic duct stone causes obstructed gallbladder ± cholecystitis

Abnormal or increased bile secretion

Pigment stones

Sterile obstruction or ascending cholangitis

Supersaturated bile
+
Nidus, e.g. bacteria
= ◯ Cholesterol stone

Common bile duct stone

Cholangitis
+ pancreatitis

Reduced bile salt recycling

Common duct stone

Causes of pancreatitis
• Abnormal pancreatic secretion, e.g. cystic fibrosis
• Gallstones
• Alcohol, drugs
• Trauma
• Mumps

Ileal disease

Bile salts

Pancreatitis

Release of enzymes, e.g. amylase, lipase, trypsin

Infection

Chronic damage to:
Pancreatic acini → Pain
+ Pancreatic insufficiency

Pancreatic islets → Diabetes mellitus

Lung damage

Tissue damage

Chronic pancreatitis

Hypoxia

Inflammation

Acute pancreatitis = severe multisystem failure

Gallstones affect up to 20% of the population in the Western world and the incidence increases with age. They may remain asymptomatic or they may cause serious illness.

Pancreatitis is often caused by passage of gallstones. It can be very severe, may become chronic and can impair pancreatic function.

Gallstones
Formation
Bile is stored in the gallbladder, where it is concentrated by epithelial cells reabsorbing water. This causes **supersaturation** of bile constituents, particularly cholesterol, which form stable **mixed micelles**

with **phospholipids** and **bile salts**. However, the supersaturated solution is unstable and cholesterol may **crystallize** around a microscopic particle or **nidus**, such as a bacterial cell. Initially crystals are very small, forming sludge or biliary sand, but they grow by accretion over time. Eighty-five percent of gallstones are **cholesterol stones**, formed in this way.

Less frequently, bile with excessively high concentrations of bile pigments is secreted, for example, in **haemolytic** diseases, such as sickle cell anaemia, causing the formation of **pigment stones**.

Ileal disease that interrupts the **entero-hepatic circulation** of bile salts, increases the risk of gallstone formation.

Pathogenesis

Most gallstones remain in the gallbladder and are **asymptomatic**, although there is a slightly increased risk of gallbladder cancer, which itself is very rare. Gallstones ejected from the gallbladder, however, may obstruct the bile ducts and are the main cause of symptomatic gallstone disease. A stone in the **cystic duct** can obstruct the gallbladder, which may then become **infected**, causing **cholecystitis**. Impacted stones in the common bile duct cause intrahepatic and extrahepatic biliary obstruction and, if the obstructed bile ducts become infected, **ascending cholangitis** results. Stones in the common bile duct or the ampulla of Vater may cause pancreatic obstruction, resulting in **pancreatitis** as well as cholangitis.

Clinical presentation

Biliary disease often causes **nausea** and **anorexia**. Symptoms may be aggravated by **fatty meals**, which stimulate cholecystokinin release, which in turn stimulates gallbladder contraction. Abdominal **pain**, localized to the **right upper quadrant**, is caused by distension of the gallbladder and bile ducts, and a tender, inflamed gallbladder may be palpable. The pain is typically **colicky**, or episodic, aggravated by waves of ineffective peristalsis. Pancreatitis and bacterial infection cause severe, persistent pain, which may be accompanied by **fever** and **rigors**.

Biliary obstruction causes **jaundice**, **pale stools**, due to absent bile pigments in the intestine, and **dark urine**, due to urinary excretion of conjugated bilirubin. Inadequate excretion of pruritogenic substances, which have not been well characterized, causes **itching**. Persistent biliary obstruction results in **malabsorption** of fats and fat-soluble vitamins due to the lack of bile salts in the intestine.

Symptoms may be **transient**, as stones can be spontaneously ejected through the sphincter of Oddi.

Diagnosis

Blood tests show raised **biliary enzymes**, **conjugated bilirubin** and inflammatory markers, such as **C-reactive protein** (see Chapter 43).

Ultrasound scanning of the abdomen sensitively detects gallstones and also shows if they are causing obstruction. Computerized tomography (**CT**) and magnetic resonance imaging (**MRI**) **scanning** may also be used (see Chapter 45).

Endoscopic retrograde cholangiopancreatography (**ERCP**) provides contrast-enhanced images of the biliary tract, demonstrating obstruction and stones in clear detail. In addition, stones can be removed endoscopically, or the sphincter of Oddi cut (**sphincterotomy**), allowing stones to pass spontaneously.

Treatment

Cholecystitis, cholangitis and pancreatitis are serious **multisystem** inflammatory disorders. Treatment includes supportive care, **analgesia** and **antibiotics**.

Gallstones are only removed when they cause clinical problems. During an episode of **acute obstruction**, infection or pancreatitis, they may be removed urgently by ERCP or surgery. More usually, the gallbladder and stones are removed surgically (**cholecystectomy**), when the acute episode has settled (see Chapter 48).

Pancreatitis

Pathogenesis

Obstruction and damage to pancreatic ducts by **stones**, **tumours or trauma** releases pancreatic enzymes that **auto-digest** duct tissue, initiating a self-perpetuating cycle of tissue damage and enzyme release that can rapidly destroy large parts of the pancreas. **Bacterial infection** and leakage of enzymes into the bloodstream often accompany this tissue damage, causing severe tissue damage at distant sites, particularly the **lungs**. Thus acute pancreatitis is a severe **multisystem disorder** that can be rapidly **fatal**.

The same mechanisms can be initiated by **chemical damage** to the pancreas caused by drugs, particularly excess **alcohol**, which is the second commonest cause of acute pancreatitis. Pancreatitis may also be caused by trauma, for example following **ERCP**, and by **infection**, for example with the mumps virus.

Clinical presentation

Abdominal **pain**, **anorexia**, **vomiting** and **fever** are the main symptoms. **Multisystem failure**, with hypotension, hypoxia and widespread intravascular haemorrhage, occurs in severe cases.

Diagnosis

Blood tests show greatly elevated circulating levels of pancreatic enzymes, particularly **amylase** and **lipase**. Inflammatory markers such as **C-reactive protein** are raised. **Hypoxia** and **hypocalcaemia** indicate severe pancreatitis. Abdominal **ultrasound** and CT or MRI scanning may demonstrate an enlarged, oedematous pancreas.

Treatment

To minimize pancreatic enzyme production, the patient is kept nil-by-mouth and the stomach is emptied by **nasogastric suction**. **Antibiotics** for presumed infection and supportive measures are the mainstay of treatment. **Specific inhibitors** of pancreatic secretion, and of pancreatic enzymes, have not yet proved clinically useful.

Chronic pancreatitis

Repeated passage of **stones** and chronic **alcohol excess** may cause recurrent pancreatitis. Inherited abnormalities in the **cystic fibrosis** gene (*CFTR*), which regulates Cl⁻ secretion in duct cells, also predisposes to chronic pancreatitis. **Repeated damage** affects **exocrine** and **endocrine** pancreatic function, causing **malabsorption** due to pancreatic enzyme deficiency and **diabetes mellitus** due to insulin deficiency. In addition, damage to sensory nerves and scarring and obstruction of the pancreatic duct cause **abdominal pain**, which can be extreme.

The scarred pancreas may develop **calcified** areas that are visible on plain abdominal X-ray.

Treatment involves replacing pancreatic enzymes with oral **supplements**, treating diabetes with **insulin** injections and **relieving pain**, which may be difficult.

41 Hepatitis and acute liver disease

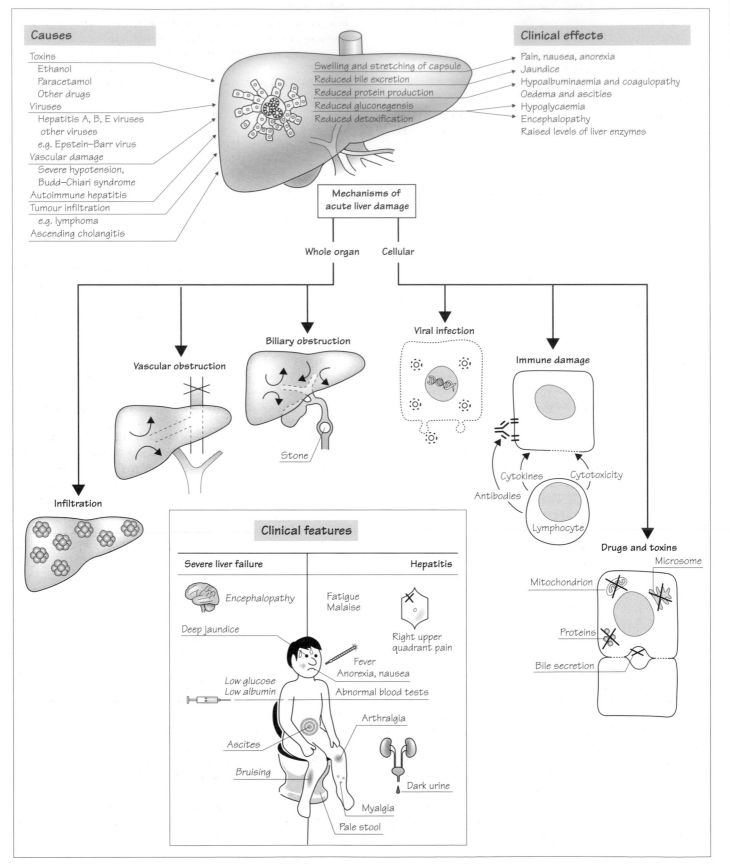

Causes

Toxins
  Ethanol
  Paracetamol
  Other drugs
Viruses
  Hepatitis A, B, E viruses
  other viruses
  e.g. Epstein–Barr virus
Vascular damage
  Severe hypotension,
  Budd–Chiari syndrome
Autoimmune hepatitis
Tumour infiltration
  e.g. lymphoma
Ascending cholangitis

Swelling and stretching of capsule
Reduced bile excretion
Reduced protein production
Reduced gluconegensis
Reduced detoxification

Clinical effects

Pain, nausea, anorexia
Jaundice
Hypoalbuminaemia and coagulopathy
Oedema and ascities
Hypoglycaemia
Encephalopathy
Raised levels of liver enzymes

Mechanisms of
acute liver damage

Whole organ   Cellular

Vascular obstruction

Biliary obstruction

Stone

Viral infection

Immune damage

Cytokines   Cytotoxicity
Antibodies
Lymphocyte

Infiltration

Drugs and toxins

Microsome
Mitochondrion
Proteins
Bile secretion

Clinical features

Severe liver failure	Hepatitis
Encephalopathy	Fatigue Malaise
Deep jaundice	Right upper quadrant pain
	Fever
	Anorexia, nausea
Low glucose Low albumin	Abnormal blood tests
	Arthralgia
Ascites	
Bruising	Dark urine
	Myalgia
	Pale stool

Hepatitis (inflammation of the liver) can occur as a result of infection, toxins, drugs and autoimmune, vascular or biliary disease. Rapidly progressive damage causes acute liver disease, while more insidious damage leads to chronic liver disease. Life-threatening **liver failure** can occur in both cases.

Viral hepatitis

Many viruses infect the liver as well as other organs, but the hepatitis viruses A, B, C, D, E and G primarily target the liver.

Hepatitis A virus is the commonest cause of viral hepatitis and, like the **hepatitis E** virus, is transmitted via the **faecal–oral** route through contaminated food or water. Infection is short-lived (about 6 weeks) and never becomes chronic, although it can be severe and even fatal. Infection induces immunity and a vaccine is available.

Hepatitis B and C viruses are transmitted by blood and sexual contact, or from mother to child. They can cause acute hepatitis, as well as **chronic hepatitis** that may progress to **cirrhosis**. In the acute phase of hepatitis B infection, patients may develop liver failure. However most develop immunity and recover, with about 10% remaining chronically infected. Acute hepatitis C infection is rarely severe, but results in chronic infection in the majority of infected individuals.

Hepatitis D virus only infects individuals with hepatitis B virus infection, which it suppresses. **Hepatitis G** virus infection is probably harmless.

The **vaccine** for hepatitis B is highly effective and there are major efforts to develop a vaccine against hepatitis C.

Drugs and toxins

The liver metabolizes drugs and toxins and is, therefore, particularly sensitive to these.

The most common liver-damaging toxin is **alcohol**, which causes metabolic damage to hepatocytes, partly by interfering with energy metabolism, resulting in **fatty liver**, and also by inducing inflammation, when it can cause **alcoholic hepatitis**. Sustained excess drinking can cause **cirrhosis**.

Some drugs and toxins (e.g. isoniazid, used to treat tuberculosis) may cause an illness resembling viral **hepatitis** and, in other cases, the **bile ducts** are targeted with little hepatocyte damage (e.g. chlorpromazine, used to treat psychosis).

Paracetamol (acetaminophen), the widely used over-the-counter analgesic, can cause massive hepatic necrosis when taken in overdose. Metabolism of paracetamol by **microsomal oxidases** generates a toxic, reactive metabolite, *N*-acetyl-*p*-benzoquinone-imine (NAPQI) that inactivates hepatocyte proteins. NAPQI is normally inactivated using **glutathione**, and hepatic stores are depleted in paracetamol overdose. *N*-acetylcysteine replenishes hepatic glutathione and therefore counteracts paracetamol toxicity (see Chapter 25).

Miscellaneous causes

Autoimmune hepatitis, characterized by reactivity against the liver, may develop in susceptible individuals, typically young women. High circulating levels of **antibodies**, some of which are directed against hepatic antigens, are typical.

Ascending cholangitis, with bacterial infection of the biliary tree and liver, may occur with biliary obstruction, caused, for example, by impacted gallstones (see Chapter 33).

Budd–Chiari syndrome is caused by obstruction of the hepatic veins, resulting in hepatic congestion and disrupted function. It is usually associated with inherited or acquired thrombophilia.

Infiltration of the liver by **tumours** can cause acute liver dysfunction and failure.

Pathogenesis

Hepatocyte damage causes accumulation of **fatty vacuoles**, and **cell death** by **necrosis** and **apoptosis**. Alcohol-induced damage causes typical **Mallory** bodies formed from precipitated intracellular proteins. In viral hepatitis, there is direct viral damage to hepatocytes, as well as **immune-mediated damage** to virally infected cells.

Inflammatory cells infiltrate the parenchyma and portal tracts. Typically, in alcoholic hepatitis, **neutrophils** predominate; while in viral hepatitis and autoimmune disease, **lymphocytes** predominate. Eosinophil-rich infiltrates characterize drug-induced liver disease. Bile duct damage causes **proliferating bile ducts** and accumulation of bile.

Clinical features

In viral hepatitis, there may be a preceding **prodromal** flu-like episode, with fever, malaise, arthralgia and myalgia. Later, **nausea, anorexia, jaundice, itching** and **abdominal pain** caused by stretching of the liver capsule develop.

Patients may develop signs of **liver failure**, including deep **jaundice**, hepatic **encephalopathy, ascites, bruising** due to decreased circulating coagulation factors, and **hypoglycaemia** due to the reduced hepatic gluconeogenesis. Liver failure is a medical **emergency** requiring urgent treatment.

Diagnosis

Liver cell damage causes increased serum levels of **transaminase enzymes** (alanine transaminase, ALT, and aspartate transaminase, AST) and damage to **biliary epithelium** raises **alkaline phosphatase** (ALP) and **γ-glutamyl transferase** (γGT) levels (see Chapter 43).

Deteriorating liver function increases the serum **bilirubin**, lowers the serum **albumin** and prolongs the **prothrombin time**, reflecting declining excretory and protein synthetic capacity (see Chapter 43).

The **cause** of acute liver damage must be determined. **Antibodies** to viruses, and circulating viral **DNA or RNA** can be measured. Circulating **paracetamol** levels can be measured and, in autoimmune hepatitis, circulating **autoantibodies** to liver antigens can be detected.

Ultrasound scan helps to determine whether the liver is chronically scarred (cirrhotic), if **vascular flow** is normal or obstructed, and if gallstones or **biliary obstruction** are present (see Chapter 45).

Treatment

Treatment is **supportive**, including nutrition, intravenous fluids and symptomatic relief of nausea and pruritis. Liver function can deteriorate rapidly and must be closely **monitored**.

Antiviral treatment. No specific treatment is available for hepatitis A or E. Hepatitis B and C infection may be treated, with partial success, using **interferon α** and antivirals such as **lamivudine** and **ribavirin**.

Autoimmune hepatitis may be treated with **corticosteroids**. Alcohol-related acute liver disease is improved by **abstinence** and alcoholic hepatitis may also require steroid treatment.

The specific antidote, *N*-acetylcysteine, should be administered early in paracetamol poisoning, before massive liver damage occurs.

Where supportive measures fail, **emergency liver transplantation** is an option. Liver function is difficult to replicate artificially and a reliable **liver support device** is not yet available.

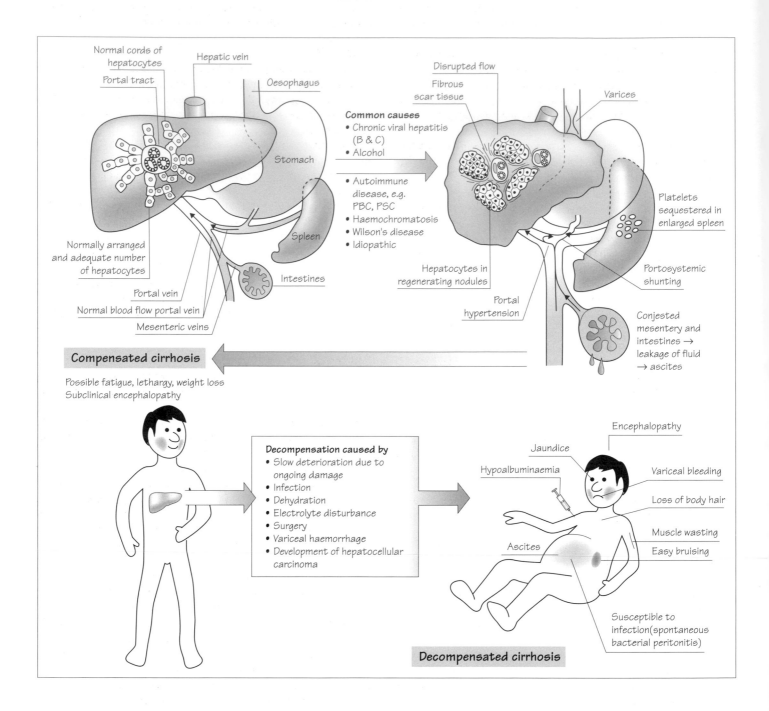

Longstanding damage to the liver eventually causes scarring and cirrhosis. Many forms of liver injury produce cirrhosis and the exact cause needs to be determined in each case to guide further treatment.

Causes

The most common causes in the Western world are excessive **alcohol** consumption, chronic **viral hepatitis** and **autoimmune liver disease**, particularly primary biliary cirrhosis (**PBC**), which affects women more frequently than men. There are many other causes, including inherited diseases such as genetic **haemochromatosis** and **Wilson's** disease (see figure above).

Multiple causes of cirrhosis can coexist and probably accelerate the rate of liver damage, for example, in people with chronic viral hepatitis or haemochromatosis who also drink alcohol.

Pathophysiology

The main effects of chronic liver damage are **reduced numbers of hepatocytes** and **disruption of the normal sinusoidal architecture**, which alters blood flow through the liver and increases pressure in the portal vein (**portal hypertension**). Haphazard regeneration of hepatocytes in nodules and formation of fibrous scar tissue by Ito (stellate) cells disrupt sinusoidal architecture (see Chapters 8 & 10). Altered blood flow further compromises liver function.

Reduced hepatic function results in the accumulation of **bilirubin** and other toxins, causing **jaundice** and itching (see Chapter 25).

As the liver is the main regulator of carbohydrate, lipid and protein **metabolism**, chronic liver disease results in widespread metabolic dysregulation, with steady weight loss and **wasting** (see Chapter 24).

The liver is the main source of circulating **plasma proteins**, including critical clotting factors, so that patients develop a tendency to bleeding (**coagulopathy**) and have reduced circulating **albumin** (see Chapter 24).

As a result of portal hypertension, **portosystemic shunting** of blood occurs where the portal and systemic venous systems meet, allowing toxin-laden blood from the intestine to bypass the liver. This contributes to chronic **hepatic encephalopathy** (also known as **portosystemic encephalopathy**), because toxic metabolites from the intestine, particularly bacterial amines, interfere with cerebral function. Shunting also promotes the development of **varices**, which can rupture and bleed catastrophically (see Chapter 10).

In addition, portal hypertension and splenic vein congestion result in **splenomegaly**, which leads to pooling of platelets in the spleen and **thrombocytopenia**. Congestion of the mesenteric veins, combined with hypoalbuminaemia can lead to transudation of fluid into the peritoneal cavity, causing **ascites**.

Clinical features

The liver has a large **functional reserve capacity**, so there may be extensive damage that remains clinically undetected, and people with cirrhosis may be totally **asymptomatic** or complain only of vague ill health and tiredness.

Eventually, however, as liver damage continues, or when an additional strain is placed on the liver, it fails to **compensate** and liver failure becomes apparent.

The effects of chronic liver disease and portal hypertension include **weight loss**, loss of **body hair**, loss of **libido**, testicular atrophy, **jaundice**, abnormal **coagulation**, **fluid** retention in the form of ankle swelling and ascites, and chronic hepatic **encephalopathy**. Hepatic encephalopathy can cause mood and sleep disturbances, a characteristic **flapping tremor** of the hands and reduced ability to perform simple mechanical tasks, such as joining dots on a page (**constructional apraxia**). Hormonal and vascular changes induce the formation of cutaneous **spider naevi**, which are arteriolar vascular malformations.

Cirrhosis may be complicated by catastrophic events, such as **variceal haemorrhage**, development of **hepatocellular carcinoma** and development of **ascites** and **infection**. Patients with ascites are at risk of developing **spontaneous bacterial peritonitis (SBP)**, caused by translocation of gram-negative bacteria from the intestinal lumen into the protein-rich ascitic fluid. This complication carries a high mortality and occurs particularly when liver disease is far advanced.

Diagnosis

Ultrasound scanning of the abdomen can detect an abnormal texture to the liver and **splenomegaly** resulting from portal hypertension. Computerized tomography (**CT**) and magnetic resonance imaging (**MRI**) **scanning** is more sensitive and can also identify portosystemic vascular shunts (see Chapter 45).

Blood tests often show abnormalities, such as raised hepatic enzyme levels, raised bilirubin, lowered albumin and abnormal coagulation tests, although all of these may be normal despite advanced cirrhosis (see Chapter 43).

Liver biopsy, showing fibrosis and regenerative hepatocyte nodules, confirms the diagnosis and may demonstrate the cause of cirrhosis, especially when special histochemical and immunohistochemical stains are used.

Blood tests can identify some causes of cirrhosis: for example autoantibodies to mitochondrial pyruvate dehydrogenase (**antimitochondrial antibodies**) indicate PBC; genetic testing for haemochromatosis is available and circulating hepatitis B DNA or hepatitis C RNA or antigen can be measured (see Chapter 41).

Treatment

Because cirrhosis is mainly **irreversible**, treatment is aimed at palliating symptoms, delaying or reducing complications, preventing further damage and avoiding liver failure.

Symptoms such as itching, weight loss and encephalopathy can be **palliated**. Itching can be treated with antihistamines and oral bile acid-binding resins, to reduce entero-hepatic recirculation.

Regular small meals with adequate calories may compensate for the loss of hepatic storage capacity, and prevent weight loss. Adequate protein intake is required to prevent muscle wasting. Chronic hepatic encephalopathy is mainly caused by portosystemic shunting rather than by hyperammonia resulting from amino acid catabolism (see Chapter 25). Encephalopathy itself is treated by laxatives, to reduce intestinal bacterial load.

Specific treatments may also be available once the cause of cirrhosis is known. For example, **antiviral** treatment may be effective for hepatitis B or C, **steroids** are effective in autoimmune hepatitis and **venesection** is used to reduce body iron stores in haemochromatosis. **Alcohol** should be avoided, to prevent further liver damage.

With advanced cirrhosis, where the risk of life-threatening complications, such as variceal haemorrhage, is high, patients may be considered for **liver transplantation**. Unfortunately, many diseases, particularly viral hepatitis, tend to recur in the transplanted liver, often at an accelerated rate.

43 Clinical assessment and blood tests

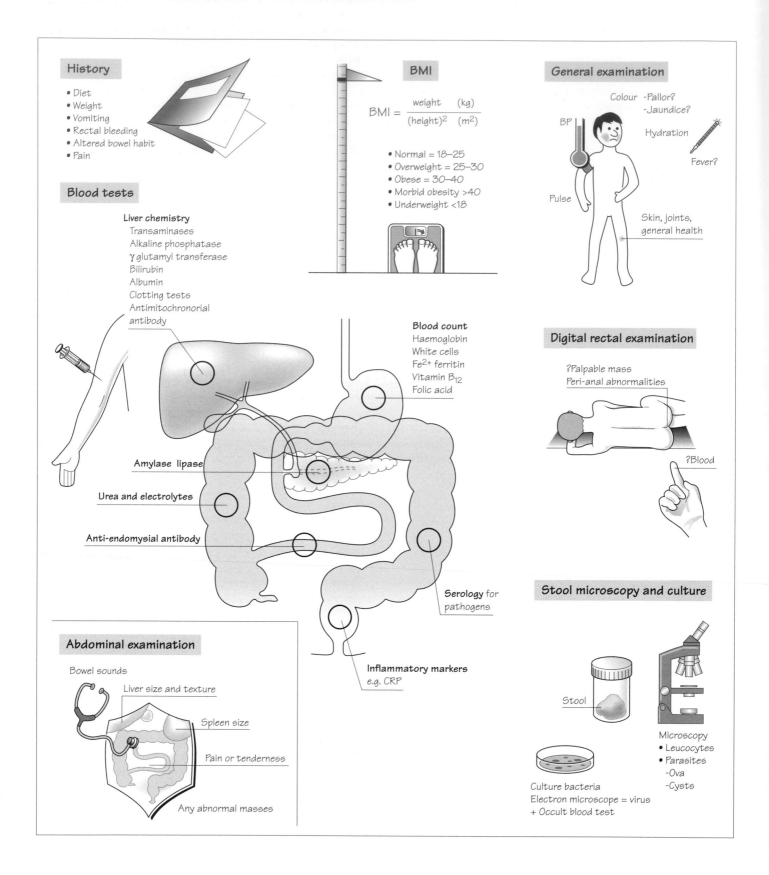

History

- Diet
- Weight
- Vomiting
- Rectal bleeding
- Altered bowel habit
- Pain

Blood tests

Liver chemistry
Transaminases
Alkaline phosphatase
γ glutamyl transferase
Bilirubin
Albumin
Clotting tests
Antimitochronorial antibody

Amylase lipase

Urea and electrolytes

Anti-endomysial antibody

BMI

$$BMI = \frac{weight \quad (kg)}{(height)^2 \quad (m^2)}$$

- Normal = 18–25
- Overweight = 25–30
- Obese = 30–40
- Morbid obesity >40
- Underweight <18

Blood count
Haemoglobin
White cells
Fe^{2+} ferritin
Vitamin B_{12}
Folic acid

Serology for pathogens

Inflammatory markers
e.g. CRP

General examination

Colour -Pallor?
        -Jaundice?
BP
Hydration
Fever?
Pulse
Skin, joints, general health

Digital rectal examination

?Palpable mass
Peri-anal abnormalities

?Blood

Abdominal examination

Bowel sounds
Liver size and texture
Spleen size
Pain or tenderness
Any abnormal masses

Stool microscopy and culture

Stool

Microscopy
- Leucocytes
- Parasites
  -Ova
  -Cysts

Culture bacteria
Electron microscope = virus
+ Occult blood test

Gastrointestinal symptoms and disorders occur frequently in clinical practice. Good clinical assessment allows one to determine how unwell the patient is and what the underlying pathological processes may be. This allows focused and effective use of endoscopy, imaging and other specialized tests.

History

- **Lifestyle**, particularly details of **diet** and **alcohol** intake must be noted, as must the use of medications, such as non-steroidal anti-inflammatory drugs (NSAIDs).
- **Travel** and potential **exposure to infection** is relevant.
- **Pain** or discomfort must be characterized and localized, and aggravating or relieving factors ascertained.
- **Altered bowel habit**, particularly of recent onset, is significant, as is recent nausea, vomiting or anorexia (loss of appetite).

Ask the patient to describe any **vomitus** and their **stool**. Does it contain blood (haematemesis or haematochezia), or is the stool black and tarry with altered blood (melaena), indicating bleeding in the upper gastrointestinal tract. Obstructive jaundice makes the stool pale and excess bile pigments darken the urine.

Any change in body weight should be noted, particularly **weight loss**, which may indicate malabsorption, chronic inflammation or cancer.

Liver, gallbladder, pancreas, stomach, small intestine and colon disorders cause vague, poorly localized symptoms. By contrast, **dysphagia** (difficulty in swallowing) usually indicates oesophageal disease.

A focused **family history** may reveal genetic predisposition to, for example, coeliac disease, inflammatory bowel disease or colorectal cancer.

Examination

Thorough general examination is mandatory, including height and weight determination and calculation of the body mass index (**BMI**). Examining the mucosae, jugular venous pressure and skin turgor helps detect **dehydration**.

The skin and sclerae should be examined for **pallor**, **jaundice** and any **rash**. **Lymphadenopathy** may indicate gastrointestinal disease; for example, Virchow's node, in the root of the neck, may indicate gastric cancer.

The abdomen should be examined with the patient lying comfortably on their back, with their arms by the side and neck and knees slightly flexed allowing the anterior abdominal wall muscles to relax. The patient should point to any area of discomfort or tenderness and this should be avoided initially during palpation.

Inspection may reveal prominent veins, herniae, visible peristalsis, protuberances or scars.

Palpation should define the position, size, texture and any tenderness of the liver, gallbladder and spleen, and any masses or lymphadenopathy.

Percussion is used to define the size and position of the liver, spleen and any masses, and to detect free fluid in the peritoneum (ascites), which shifts when the patient's position is altered (shifting dullness).

Auscultation is used to assess bowel sounds. In paralytic ileus they are absent, while in intestinal obstruction they may be increased.

Genitalia and digital rectal examination: inspect the external genitalia, inguinal hernial orifices and peri-anal region. For the digital rectal examination, the patient lies on their left-hand side, with their drawn up. The peri-anal skin should be inspected and palpated gloved, lubricated finger inserted gently into the anus, assessin tone and feeling for any abnormal masses or swellings. The with gloved finger should be inspected to detect bleeding.

Stool examination

Volume, consistency, colour and the presence of fat globules, indicating malabsorption, should be noted. True diarrhoea implies an increased stool volume, above 200–300 mL/day.

Microscopy is used to detect parasites, ova or cysts and leucocytes or pus cells, which occur in dysentery or intestinal inflammation. **Electron microscopy** can be used to detect viral infection and stool **culture** to identify bacterial pathogens. Toxins can be detected by special tests.

Chemical testing can be used to detect small amounts of blood that are macroscopically invisible (**faecal occult blood**). This may indicate intestinal bleeding, although dietary haem and enzymes can cause false positive reactions.

Basic blood tests

- **Blood count**. Anaemia may indicate many serious gastrointestinal diseases, such as peptic ulcer, malabsorption and intestinal cancer. The platelet count, white cell count and red cell indices, as well as levels of iron, ferritin, vitamin B_{12} and folic acid, may be abnormal in malabsorption, inflammatory bowel disease and liver disease.
- **Clotting tests**. A prolonged prothrombin time (PT) may indicate synthetic liver failure or vitamin K deficiency, for example, caused by malabsorption of fat-soluble vitamins.
- **Urea and electrolytes**. Intestinal bleeding causes increased amino acid absorption and, therefore, increases the amount of urea produced by the liver. Urea and electrolyte levels may also indicate dehydration, or renal damage. Calcium levels may be reduced in malabsorption.
- **Liver chemistry**. The serum **albumin** level is reduced in liver failure, as part of the acute phase response caused by inflammation, and in malnutrition.

Alanine and aspartate **transaminase** (ALT and AST) levels are raised by liver cell damage and the **alkaline phosphatase** (ALP) and γ-**glutamyl transferase** (γGT) levels are increased in biliary tract disease. γGT levels are also raised by excess alcohol consumption.

Bilirubin levels are increased in liver and biliary disease. Jaundice is clinically readily apparent when bilirubin levels are raised two- to threefold.

- **Inflammatory markers**. Increased levels of C-reactive protein (CRP) and a raised erythrocyte sedimentation rate (ESR) may indicate inflammatory bowel disease (IBD), acute pancreatitis or infection.
- **Amylase and lipase levels**. Acute pancreatitis causes massively raised amylase or lipase levels and more modestly increased levels are seen in conditions such as peptic ulcer.
- **Serological tests**. Exquisitely sensitive and specific serological tests can be used to diagnose coeliac disease (antibodies to tissue transglutaminase) and primary biliary cirrhosis (antimitochondrial antibody). Circulating autoantibodies are also found in atrophic gastritis and autoimmune hepatitis. Serological tests for hepatitis viruses and gastrointestinal infections, such as amoebiasis, are also available.

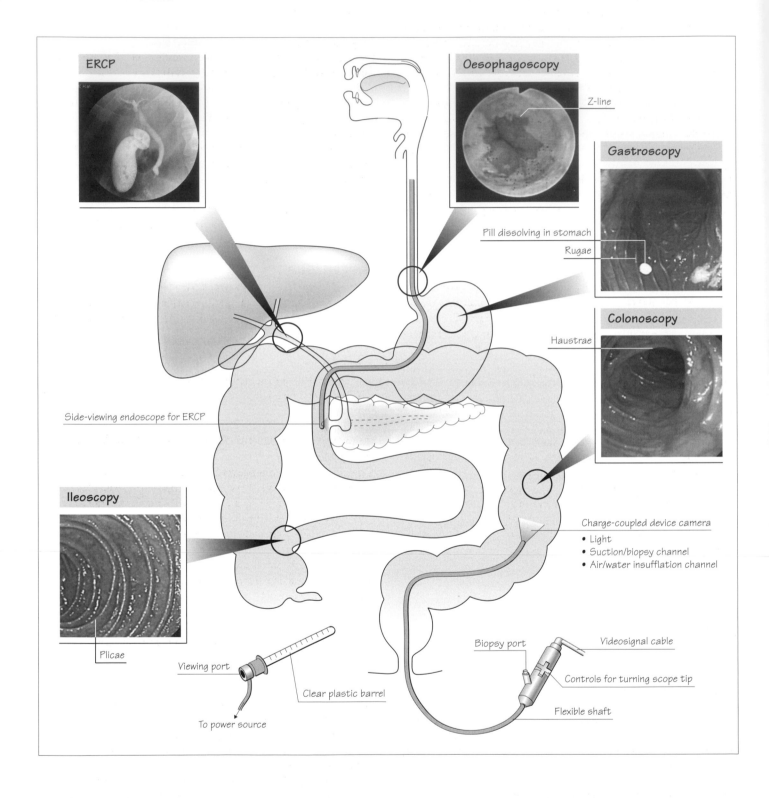

Direct visualization of the interior of the hollow gastrointestinal organs is one of the most powerful diagnostic and therapeutic modalities in modern medicine. The earliest endoscopes were rigid instruments, allowing visualization along a straight line. **Fibreoptic** instruments, which transmit light around curves, extended the range of endoscopy.

Modern video endoscopes use a **charge-coupled device**, or an electronic camera, to capture and transmit images electronically, so there is no optical limit to their movement. Most instruments have channels for insufflation and suction and to introduce instruments, such as forceps, for taking biopsies.

Rigid instruments

These are stainless steel or plastic tubes with a light source and a single channel for observation and instrumentation.

The **rigid sigmoidoscope** can be inserted up to 20 cm into the rectum and proximal sigmoid colon, and is routinely used to diagnose proctitis and rectal tumours. The shorter and wider **proctoscope** allows examination of the anal canal and rectum. Haemorrhoids can be treated by sclerotherapy or elastic band ligation through a proctoscope.

Rigid **oesophagogastroscopes** are now mainly used to treat oesophageal obstruction caused by foreign bodies, such as food boluses, because the wide channel allows rapid removal or displacement of the obstruction.

Flexible upper gastrointestinal endoscopy

The oesophagus, stomach and proximal duodenum are routinely visualized and the distal duodenum and jejunum may occasionally be seen.

Diagnostic uses

Investigation of heartburn, dyspepsia and occult blood loss are the commonest indications. **Biopsies** can be taken to diagnose *Helicobacter pylori* infection, inflammation or neoplasia. Plastic **brushes** can be rubbed along lesions, capturing superficial cells or pathogens to diagnose cancer and infection. Jejunal fluid can be **aspirated** and examined for pathogens such as *Giardia lamblia*.

Therapeutic uses

The commonest lesions treated endoscopically are **bleeding peptic ulcers**, which can be injected with epinephrine (adrenaline) to cause vasospasm, and **ruptured oesophageal varices**, which can be injected with sclerosant or ligated with rubber bands to halt bleeding and cause fibrosis and subsequent obliteration. Other bleeding lesions may be treated using lasers or electrocautery.

Obstruction caused either by gastro-oesophageal tumours or by benign strictures can be relieved by **dilatation** using balloon or rigid dilators, and plastic or metal **stents** can then be introduced to maintain patency of the lumen. Pneumatic **dilatation** or endoscopic injection of **botulinum toxin** into the lower oesophageal sphincter may relieve obstruction caused by achalasia.

Complications

Upper endoscopy itself is relatively safe and can be performed with or without light **sedation** of the patient. Therapy such as dilatation may cause rupture of the oesophagus.

Enteroscopy

Long, thin instruments with a rigid outer casing that straightens the shaft proximally can be introduced into the jejunum and ileum. The tip of a **Sonde** enteroscope is propelled by peristalsis and can reach the distal small intestine. Unfortunately, the distance either instrument has progressed cannot be reliably ascertained and biopsies cannot be taken with Sonde enteroscopes.

Colonoscopy and flexible sigmoidoscopy

Fibreoptic and video colonoscopes allow examination of the entire **large intestine** and the **terminal ileum**. The patient must be adequately prepared beforehand with powerful **laxatives** to remove solid material from the colon. During the examination, light **sedation** and **analgesia** are usually necessary. In flexible sigmoidoscopy the instrument is only inserted into the left side of the colon.

Diagnostic uses

The commonest indications include investigation of **altered bowel habit**, **rectal bleeding**, suspected **colorectal cancer** and **inflammatory bowel disease**. Colonoscopic screening for colon cancer is advocated for patients at high risk, for example, those with a strong family history of the disease, and there is a debate about introducing population-wide screening.

The normal colonic mucosa is smooth and shiny with a regular vascular pattern. Pouches or **diverticulae** can be easily detected, as can inflamed, ulcerated or bleeding areas, **polyps** and malignant **tumours**. **Biopsies** for histology can safely be taken and polyps and small tumours removed by **snaring** and **electrocautery**.

Ileoscopy: the tip of the colonoscope can be manoeuvred through the ileocaecal valve into the terminal ileum.

Therapeutic uses

Bleeding lesions can be treated by **electrocautery** or heat coagulation and small polyps removed (**polypectomy**). Large tumours causing bleeding or obstruction can be treated with **lasers**, and **stents** introduced to maintain a patent lumen.

Complications

There is a small risk of colonic **perforation**, and of **bleeding** following polypectomy. Sedation and analgesia may also cause **respiratory depression**.

Endoscopic retrograde cholangiopancreatography and biliary endoscopy

A duodenoscope with a sideways-facing tip allows visualization and cannulation of the **ampulla of Vater**. **Contrast material** can then be injected into the pancreatic and biliary ducts and **X-ray images** taken. Close-up **ultrasound** images can be obtained by inserting compact ultrasound probes into the duct. Cannulae and instruments can be introduced to obtain **brushings** or **biopsies**, remove **gallstones**, and dilate strictures. The sphincter of Oddi may be cut (**sphincterotomy**), allowing gallstones to pass spontaneously.

Endoscopic retrograde cholangiopancreatography (**ERCP**) is usually performed to investigate and treat obstructive jaundice. Larger bile ducts can also be viewed with very fine flexible endoscopes inserted percutaneously into the liver. Injecting contrast material into the pancreatic duct can provoke **pancreatitis**.

Future directions

Advanced instruments are making endoscopy safer and more versatile. Ingeniously designed instruments that can be inserted alongside the endoscope or through the biopsy channel are expanding the range of therapeutic interventions to include **cutting** and **suturing**, enabling **endoscopic surgery**.

Wireless capsule endoscopy: tiny encapsulated electronic cameras can be swallowed, allowing visual data be collected remotely, by **radio transmission**. Images are thus obtained from areas that cannot be reached by conventional endoscopic instruments, although biopsies cannot yet be taken.

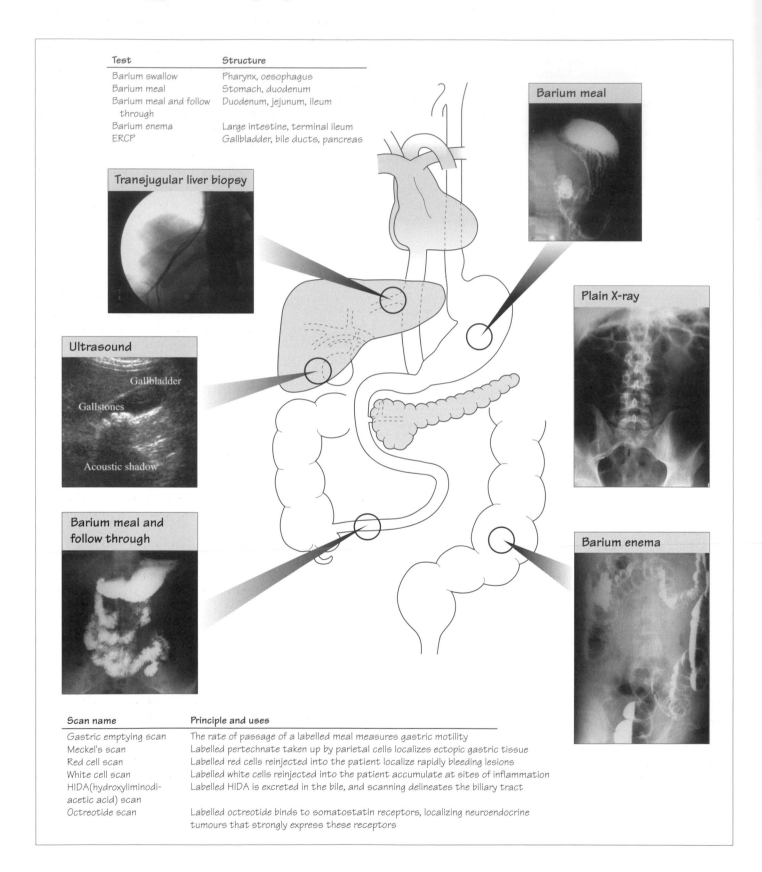

Test	Structure
Barium swallow	Pharynx, oesophagus
Barium meal	Stomach, duodenum
Barium meal and follow through	Duodenum, jejunum, ileum
Barium enema	Large intestine, terminal ileum
ERCP	Gallbladder, bile ducts, pancreas

Transjugular liver biopsy

Barium meal

Ultrasound

Gallbladder

Gallstones

Acoustic shadow

Plain X-ray

Barium meal and follow through

Barium enema

Scan name	Principle and uses
Gastric emptying scan	The rate of passage of a labelled meal measures gastric motility
Meckel's scan	Labelled pertechnate taken up by parietal cells localizes ectopic gastric tissue
Red cell scan	Labelled red cells reinjected into the patient localize rapidly bleeding lesions
White cell scan	Labelled white cells reinjected into the patient accumulate at sites of inflammation
HIDA(hydroxyliminodi-acetic acid) scan	Labelled HIDA is excreted in the bile, and scanning delineates the biliary tract
Octreotide scan	Labelled octreotide binds to somatostatin receptors, localizing neuroendocrine tumours that strongly express these receptors

X-rays, ultrasound scanning, magnetic resonance imaging (MRI) and isotope scanning are powerful techniques for investigating structure and function in the gastrointestinal system and can also be used therapeutically.

Plain X-rays

There is little intrinsic difference in radio-opacity, or contrast, between most intra-abdominal structures, which makes plain abdominal X-rays challenging to interpret. Nonetheless, they can be rapidly and cheaply performed and help to diagnose a number of common conditions. For example, excess gas and fluid accumulate in **intestinal obstruction**, creating multiple air–fluid levels, and in severe **colitis**, colonic dilatation may create an enlarged gas-filled colon (**toxic megacolon**) that is readily visualized. Free air in the peritoneum is detected in **intestinal perforation** and pancreatic calcification is visible in **chronic pancreatitis**. **Colonic transit** time can be simply determined by sequentially ingesting radio-opaque shapes and performing plain X-rays at intervals thereafter (**shape test**).

Plain X-rays with luminal contrast

X-ray contrast material can be administered orally, instilled rectally or injected endoscopically to delineate the interior of the intestinal tract and demonstrate **ulcers**, **strictures**, **diverticulae**, **fistulae** and **tumours**. **Fluoroscopic real-time** views of the passage of contrast allow **peristalsis** and functional abnormalities of, for example, swallowing, oesophageal and gastric emptying, and defecation to be investigated. The most frequently used contrast agents are **barium**, and **gastrograffin**, which is more water-soluble. Striking double-contrast images of the mucosal surface are obtained by instilling air with the liquid contrast. Common specific tests are shown in the table in the figure.

Computerized tomography scan

Cross-sectional images produced by computerized tomography (CT) scanning effectively image the **liver**, **gallbladder** and **pancreas**. It is less useful for imaging the hollow organs, although new techniques, using increased computing power, allow three-dimensional reconstruction of the colon, providing high-resolution **virtual colonoscopy** with contrast provided by luminal insufflation of air or CO_2.

CT scanning can also be enhanced by oral or rectal **contrast**, delineating the bowel lumen or by intravenous contrast, which increases the definition of **vascular structures** in the liver, pancreas and bowel wall.

Magnetic resonance imaging

The resolution of magnetic resonance imaging (MRI) scans is generally greater than that of CT scans and intravenous **gadolinium**, which is a magnetic contrast agent, further enhances the definition of vascular structures. With powerful computer algorithms that analyze the effect of blood or bile flow on the image, magnetic resonance angiography (**MRA**) and magnetic resonance cholangiopancreatography (**MRCP**) allow reconstruction of the vascular and biliary anatomy, and may replace conventional vascular angiography and endoscopic retrograde cholangiopancreatography (ERCP) in some cases. Thus MRI scanning, which does not involve harmful radiation, is rapidly becoming a major imaging modality in gastroenterology.

Ultrasound scanning

Ultrasound scanning (USS) is particularly useful for examining the liver and gallbladder. USS detects 90% of **gallstones** (compared to 10% detected by X-rays) and can also be used to evaluate the texture of the liver, the thickness of the **gallbladder** wall and the calibre of **bile ducts**. USS can also image the pancreas although overlying bowel gas makes this unreliable. Free fluid in the peritoneum, or **ascites**, is also readily demonstrated by USS. It is less helpful for examining air-filled structures, such as the intestinal tract.

Using **Doppler** measurements, the rate and direction of blood flow in the portal and hepatic veins can be determined, which is useful in **portal hypertension** and the **Budd–Chiari** syndrome.

An ultrasound probe inserted into the anal canal (**endoanal USS**) can provide high-resolution images of the sphincter muscles and surrounding tissues, helping to evaluate the depth of anorectal inflammation or neoplasia. **Endoscopic USS** probes in the oesophagus, stomach, duodenum and ampulla of Vater to produce similarly close-up images of the walls of these structures.

Radioisotope scans

Gamma-ray emitting isotopes can be attached to various molecules that localize to different body compartments and their distribution detected with a gamma ray detector. For example, isotopes can be attached to **monoclonal antibodies** with exquisite specificity for their target proteins, allowing localization of rare tumours and cells. This can also be used to target high-dose local **radiotherapy**. Thus, the technique is versatile, although it provides relatively low anatomical resolution. Various radioisotope scans are listed in the table in the figure.

Positron emission tomography (PET) detects the abnormal accumulation of labelled compounds, such as glucose in metabolically active cells, and can localize tumours and inflammation with greater sensitivity and spatial resolution than conventional radioisotope scanning.

Interventional radiology

Radiological guidance with USS, CT or MRI, enables invasive procedures, such as a liver biopsy, to be performed more safely and with greater precision.

X-ray fluoroscopy can guide **dilatation** of strictures and placement of **stents** in, for example, the oesophagus, and allows vascular manipulations, such as **embolization** of bleeding vessels in the intestinal tract. Similarly, liver tumours can be treated by X-ray guided embolization of the arterial supply, as the portal vein continues to supply blood to the surrounding liver.

Liver biopsies can be taken by passing forceps **transjugularly** into the hepatic vein under fluoroscopic guidance, avoiding the bleeding risk associated with percutaneous biopsy. Similarly, a shunt between the hepatic vein and portal vein can be created transjugularly, under fluoroscopic guidance, to relieve portal hypertension and associated bleeding varices. This is known as a transjugular intrahepatic portosystemic shunt (**TIPSS**).

Insufflating air and barium into the colon during a barium enema may suffice to reduce and treat **volvulus** of the sigmoid colon. Similarly, increased luminal pressure created by a barium enema can reduce **intussusception**, where a proximal part of the intestine is drawn into the distal lumen by peristalsis.

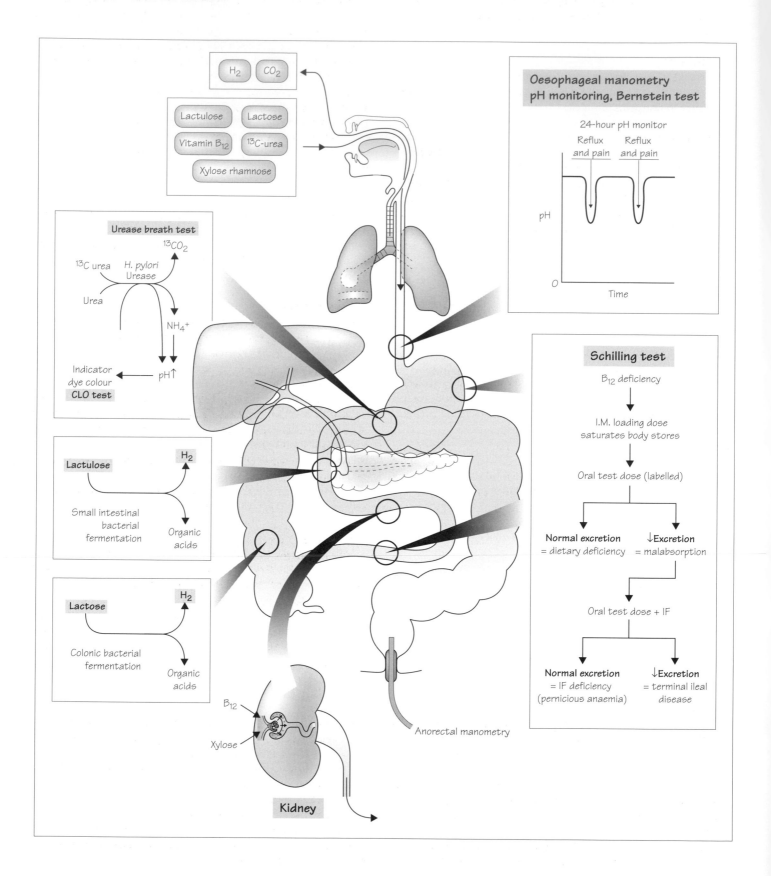

Oesophageal manometry
pH monitoring, Bernstein test

24-hour pH monitor

Reflux and pain

Schilling test

B_{12} deficiency

I.M. loading dose
saturates body stores

Oral test dose (labelled)

Normal excretion
= dietary deficiency

↓Excretion
= malabsorption

Oral test dose + IF

Normal excretion
= IF deficiency
(pernicious anaemia)

↓Excretion
= terminal ileal
disease

Urease breath test

$^{13}CO_2$

^{13}C urea
H. pylori
Urease

Urea

NH_4^+

Indicator
dye colour

pH↑

CLO test

Lactulose

H_2

Small intestinal
bacterial
fermentation

Organic
acids

Lactose

H_2

Colonic bacterial
fermentation

Organic
acids

H_2 CO_2

Lactulose   Lactose

Vitamin B_{12} ^{13}C-urea

Xylose rhamnose

B_{12}

Xylose

Kidney

Anorectal manometry

Functional tests measure aspects of gastrointestinal pathophysiology and complement endoscopy, radiological imaging and blood tests. There are many specific tests available and some of the underlying principles are discussed here.

Breath tests

The principle underlying these tests is that gases such as CO_2 and H_2 that can be generated in the intestine are rapidly absorbed into the circulation and excreted through the lungs.

^{13}C-urease breath test

This test detects the presence of the urease enzyme of *Helicobacter pylori* in the stomach. A drink containing ^{13}C-labelled urea is administered and, after a short interval, a sample of expiratory breath is taken to detect the presence of ^{13}C-labelled CO_2, produced by the breakdown of ^{13}C- urea, principally by the urease enzyme of *H. pylori*. ^{13}C is a non-radioactive isotope and it is measured by mass spectrometry; similar tests use ^{14}C-labelled urea, which emits beta particles that are detected by scintigraphy.

Lactose breath test

A test meal containing lactose is administered and the amount of H_2 excreted on the breath is measured over the subsequent few hours. Normally lactose is digested in the intestine by the enzyme lactase and absorbed, resulting in no excess production of H_2. However, in **lactase deficiency**, either congenital, or acquired, for example after a bout of gastroenteritis, lactose passes undigested into the large intestine, where bacteria metabolize it, releasing H_2. The excess H_2 is absorbed into the bloodstream and excreted via the lungs.

Lactulose breath test

Lactulose is a disaccharide that is not absorbed or metabolized in the small intestine and passes to the colon, where bacteria digest it, releasing H_2. H_2 is produced after a delay necessitated by the passage of lactulose through the small intestine. However, where there is **bacterial overgrowth** in the small intestine, lactulose metabolism occurs in the small intestine and is accelerated, resulting in excessive and early H_2 production.

Absorption and excretion tests

The principle underlying these tests is that tracer compounds absorbed from the intestine can be readily detected in the bloodstream or in the urine when they are excreted. The chosen tracer compounds are easily detected, either by measuring radioactivity, or by a simple chemical test.

Schilling test

This test investigates the various steps in the absorption of vitamin B_{12} (hydroxocobalamin).

Firstly, a large dose of vitamin B_{12} is administered by intramuscular injection, to saturate body stores and ensure that any additional vitamin B_{12} that is absorbed will be excreted in the urine rather than stored.

Next an oral dose of radiolabelled vitamin B_{12} is administered and the urinary excretion measured. Providing that intestinal absorption is normal, most of the labelled vitamin will be detected in the urine, suggesting that any previous deficiency was due to dietary insufficiency.

If, however, excretion cannot be detected, implying that there is inadequate intestinal absorption, a further oral dose of radiolabelled vitamin B_{12} is administered, this time together with intrinsic factor (IF). If exogenous IF restores normal absorption and excretion, the interpretation is that the patient has pernicious anaemia, or IF deficiency caused by atrophic gastritis.

If, however, exogenous IF fails to restore normal absorption and excretion, the likely cause of vitamin B_{12} deficiency is disease of, or damage to, the terminal ileum.

Bromsulpthalein excretion test

Bromsulpthalein administered orally is almost entirely taken up by the liver and excreted in the bile. If there is reduced hepatic function, or altered biliary excretion, an increased proportion of bromsulpthalcin is excreted in the urine.

Xylose excretion

Xylose is a non-metabolized sugar that is absorbed in the small intestine. Once absorbed into the bloodstream, it is excreted unchanged in the urine. Thus urinary excretion allows intestinal absorption and permeability to be measured. The xylose excretion test is mainly used as a research tool.

Stimulation tests

In these tests a hormone or other physiological stimulus is administered and the response noted. In most cases this involves measuring the secretion of another hormone or chemical into the circulation.

Secretin test

This test is used to assess the extent of functional pancreatic tissue. The **duodenum** is intubated and secretin infused intravenously. The amount of pancreatic juice secreted and the HCO_3^- **concentration** and content is measured. These are directly correlated with the amount of functional pancreatic tissue and low levels indicate **pancreatic insufficiency** caused, for example, by chronic pancreatitis.

The test can be augmented by also infusing **cholecystokinin** and measuring pancreatic **enzyme** secretion.

Manometry

Pressure transducers introduced into parts of the intestinal tract allow the function of sphincters to be studied. The most commonly performed measurements are of the lower **oesophageal** and **anal** sphincters and the **sphincter of Oddi**.

Oesophageal manometry is used to diagnose various dysmotility disorders, including diffuse oesophageal spasm and achalasia of the cardia, while anal manometry helps in the diagnosis of the causes of faecal incontinence.

pH measurement

pH electrodes introduced into the oesophagus and stomach through the nose or mouth allow the frequency and severity of gastro-oesophageal acid reflux to be evaluated. Episodes of low pH in the distal oesophagus are correlated with symptoms, to ensure that reflux **symptoms** are actually caused by acid reflux. The test can be used to document the effects of medical and surgical treatment.

In the **Bernstein test**, dilute HCl may be infused into the lower oesophagus, to determine if this reproduces heartburn for the patient.

Oesophageal pH measurement can be performed in ambulatory patients, over a 24-h period, allowing documentation of the effects of meals, posture and sleeping.

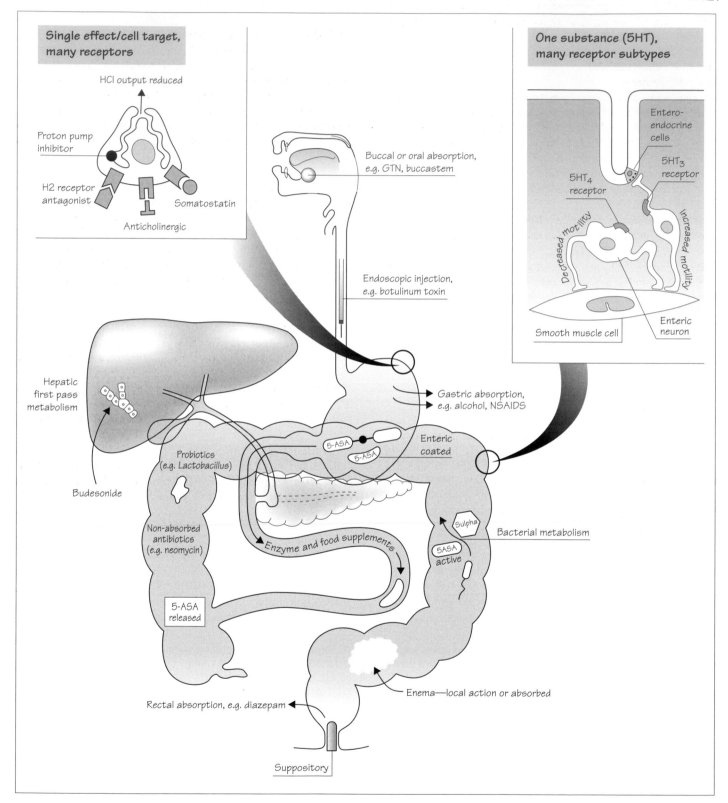

Single effect/cell target, many receptors

HCl output reduced

Proton pump inhibitor

H2 receptor antagonist

Somatostatin

Anticholinergic

One substance (5HT), many receptor subtypes

Entero-endocrine cells

5HT₃ receptor

5HT₄ receptor

Decreased motility

Increased motility

Smooth muscle cell

Enteric neuron

Buccal or oral absorption, e.g. GTN, buccastem

Endoscopic injection, e.g. botulinum toxin

Gastric absorption, e.g. alcohol, NSAIDS

Hepatic first pass metabolism

Budesonide

Probiotics (e.g. Lactobacillus)

5-ASA

5-ASA

Enteric coated

Non-absorbed antibiotics (e.g. neomycin)

Enzyme and food supplements

Sulpha

5ASA active

Bacterial metabolism

5-ASA released

Enema—local action or absorbed

Rectal absorption, e.g. diazepam

Suppository

Pharmacological treatment of gastrointestinal disorders is a mature and well-advanced field, and new treatments are constantly emerging. The largest selling drugs recently have been gastrointestinal acid suppressants, reflecting the high incidence of dyspepsia and peptic ulceration and the exquisite specificity of the medications with the resulting low incidence of adverse effects.

Special considerations

Target specificity

Many drugs bind to cellular receptors or proteins selectively. By mimicking the structure of the naturally occurring chemical, its effect is either replicated (agonist) or blocked (antagonist). An example is the group of histamine H2 receptor antagonists that block acid secretion by parietal cells. With advancing scientific knowledge, greater specificity can be achieved: for example different serotonin (5-hydroxytryptamine, 5HT) receptor subtypes are now being selectively targeted.

Selective release and topical treatment

Another way of achieving selective effects is to only apply the medication where it can reach the target tissue. In the gastrointestinal system, this can be achieved by oral administration of non-absorbed drugs that then act locally. The 5-aminosalicylic acid (5ASA, mesalazine) drugs used to treat inflammatory bowel disease (IBD) are delivered this way, either as slow-release preparations that dissolve in the distal intestine or as pro-drugs that are activated by bacterial metabolism in the colon.

Some drugs are significantly absorbed through the rectal mucosa, such as diazepam, used to treat active epileptic fitting, while others, such as rectal 5ASA compounds, act locally.

Hepatic first pass effect

Enterically administered drugs that are rapidly and completely metabolized by the liver are said to have high hepatic first pass metabolism. This allows high doses to be delivered to the intestine, with fewer systemic side-effects. An example is the synthetic corticosteroid, **budesonide**, used to treat IBD.

Augmenting or inhibiting intestinal function

Pancreatic enzyme supplements and lactase can be taken by mouth to correct the effects of pancreatic failure and intestinal hypolactasia, respectively. The enzyme supplements act locally in the intestine. Orlistat, which is designed to reduce fat absorption, acts by inhibiting pancreatic lipase in the intestine.

Oral tolerance, immunotherapy and vaccination

Orally administered antigens stimulate a strong secretory immune response with immunoglobulin A (IgA) and IgM antibodies, while the systemic immune response is inhibited. Thus the live polio vaccine and vaccines against salmonellae and *Vibrio cholera* are administered orally. Orally administered autoantigens may induce selective immunological tolerance and could be used to treat autoimmune diseases, such as multiple sclerosis, although results of clinical trials have so far been discouraging.

Antibiotics and probiotics

Some intestinal symptoms may be due to a proliferation of abnormal intestinal bacteria or reduced normal commensals, and oral or rectal administration of live commensal bacteria is currently being investigated, particularly in the treatment of IBD. This is a counterpart to the administration of **antibiotics** to **selectively decontaminate** the intestinal lumen, for example, before abdominal surgery or in chronic liver disease.

Food as therapy

Intolerance to various food elements occurs, for example, in coeliac disease, lactose intolerance, cow's milk protein, peanut and other food allergies.

A totally bland, antigen-free diet comprising monomers or short oligomers of carbohydrate, fat and protein is apparently effective in treating Crohn's disease, although the mechanism of action is unknown.

Enteral feeding

Enteral, as opposed to parenteral, **feeding**, even in severely ill patients is critically important, as the food-free intestine atrophies, increasing the risk of bacterial translocation and systemic sepsis.

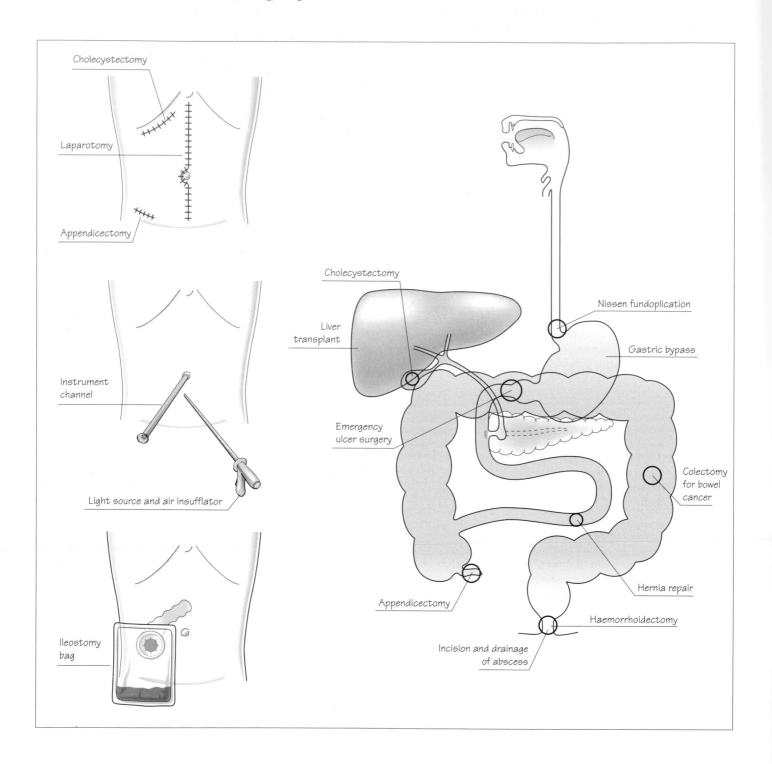

Incision of the abdominal wall to gain access to the peritoneal cavity is termed **laparotomy**. **Minimally invasive laparoscopic surgery** has transformed many abdominal operations from major, hazardous undertakings, to routine day-case procedures. However, gastrointestinal surgery is frequently performed as an **emergency** and remains highly demanding for the patient and surgeon.

In addition, many gastrointestinal disorders are treated jointly by physicians and surgeons, who collaborate to determine the best combined therapeutic approach for individual patients, particularly when managing inflammatory bowel disease (IBD) and hepatobiliary conditions.

Basic considerations

As for any surgery performed under general anaesthetic, patients fast beforehand and, for intestinal surgery, the bowel is also **purged** with laxatives, and prophylactic **antibiotics** are administered peri-operatively.

Manipulating the intestine temporarily halts peristalsis, causing **paralytic ileus**; therefore, patients cannot eat or drink immediately after abdominal surgery.

Stomas

Parts of the intestinal tract are commonly brought out onto the surface of the abdomen, creating an artificial opening or stoma. This may be **permanent** or **temporary**, allowing time for the distal part of the bowel to heal, or to **defunction** the distal intestine prior to further surgery.

Stomas release intestinal or colonic contents onto the skin, which is not adapted for constant exposure to their pH, salt and enzymatic composition; therefore, stomas require special care, involving equipment such as adhesive dressings and bags.

In addition, small intestinal stomas lose large volumes of intestinal juice that can no longer be reabsorbed by the colon and patients risk **salt and water depletion** unless they compensate by increasing intake.

Laparoscopic surgery

Operations such as a **cholecystectomy** are now usually performed laparoscopically whereby instead of a large incision of the anterior abdominal wall, a small 'keyhole' incision is made through which a narrow laparoscope is inserted. This allows visualization of the internal organs and instruments are introduced through the same or additional incisions to perform the surgery. The technique requires skill and practice and is much less traumatic for the patient.

Common operations

- **Cholecystectomy**: usually to remove symptomatic gallstones causing cholangitis or pancreatitis.
- **Hernia repair**: such as inguinal hernias, particularly in men.
- **Appendicectomy**: usually for acute appendicitis.

Gastrointestinal bleeding

Fifty per cent of gastrointestinal bleeding is caused by **peptic ulcers** and, although many cases can be treated medically or endoscopically, uncontrollable bleeding, especially where the bleeding source cannot be identified, necessitates **emergency laparotomy**.

Gastrointestinal bleeding caused by portal hypertension may require surgically constructed vascular shunts (**portocaval shunts**) to reduce portal pressure and prevent variceal haemorrhage.

Inflammatory bowel disease

Inflammatory bowel disease, particularly Crohn's disease, can cause intestinal **strictures** and **fistulae** that require surgical correction. However, as Crohn's disease typically recurs after surgery, surgery is used sparingly.

Medically uncontrolled colitis may necessitate emergency **colectomy** as a life-saving measure. Furthermore, in ulcerative colitis, colectomy is **curative** and is sometimes also performed because of the high risk of **colorectal cancer**.

Cancer

Cancers of the intestinal tract, pancreas, liver or gallbladder may be treated surgically, particularly if they are detected at an early, potentially curable stage. However, most operations are palliative, aiming to reduce tumour bulk before chemotherapy or radiotherapy, or to relieve intestinal obstruction or bleeding.

Obesity

Surgical treatment of obesity is still evolving. The earliest operations, in which the jejunum and varying lengths of ileum were **bypassed**, achieved weight loss but were complicated by steatohepatitis causing severe liver damage, and are no longer performed.

Wiring the jaws closed, so that the patient cannot eat solid food and must subsist on liquids is effective. **Gastroplication** reduces the effective size of the gastric reservoir, forcing patients to eat smaller meals.

Transplantation

Transplant surgery may be performed to replace the **liver**, **pancreas** or pancreatic islet tissue, or **small intestine**. Orthotopic liver transplantion, whereby the original liver is removed and replaced with a donor organ is the most successful, and 85% of liver transplant recipients survive for at least 5 years post-operatively. Pancreatic and small intestinal transplantation are less successful, although when the small intestine and liver are transplanted together, the outcome improves, possibly because liver transplantation induces **donor-specific immune tolerance** in the host, reducing the risk of rejection.

Index

Note: page numbers in *italics* refer to figures

tonsils *12*, 13, 17
  immune function *46*, 47
total parenteral nutrition (TPN) 55
touch sensation 45
toxic megacolon 101
toxins 77
  shunting 31
tractus solitarius *16*, 17, 45
transaminases *58*, 59, 93, *96*, 97
transcobalamin *52*, 53
transcytosis *46*, 47
transferrin *52*, 53
transforming growth factor β (TGFβ) 43
transjugular intrahepatic portosystemic shunt
    (TIPSS) *30*, 31, *100*, 101
transplant surgery 107
  liver 93, 95, 107
transporter proteins *28*, 29
  genetic abnormalities 51
trefoil proteins *36*, 37
tremor, flapping 95
tri-radiate fold *34*, 35
tricyclic antidepressants 69
trigeminal nerve *12*, 13, 17
triglycerides 49, *50*, 51
Tropheryma whippelii 77
tropical sprue 33, *76*, 77, 81
trypsin *50*, 51
trypsinogen *50*, 51
tuberculosis 35, 75, 77
  ileocaecal 33
two-hit and multiple gene theory 85
typhoid fever 33, 75

ulcerative colitis 35, 37, 39, *78*, 79
  environmental triggers 77, *78*, 79
  proctitis 89
  treatment 79
ulcers, apthous 13, *78*, 79
ultrasound imaging 99, *100*, 101
undernutrition *see* nutritional deficiency
uraemia 17
urea
  excretion 55, 61
  levels 97
urea cycle *60*, 61

urease breath test 73
urine, urea excretion 61

vaccination 105
vagotomy 21
  selective *72*, 73
vagus nerve 17, *18*, 19, *20*, 21
  dysfunction 69
  foregut/midgut innervation *44*, 45
  pancreas innervation *24*, 25
  peptic ulcer surgery *72*, 73
valves of Houston *38*, 39
varices *30*, 31
  cirrhosis 95
  see also oesophageal varices
vascular structure CT contrast imaging 101
vasoactive intestinal peptide (VIP) *42*, 43, 57
  neuro-endocrine tumour production *86*,
    87
vasoactive intestinal peptide (VIP)-secreting
    tumours 43, 57, *64*, 65
vasopressin 57
vegans 53
venesection 95
vermillion border of lips *12*, 13
Verner–Morrison syndrome 87
very low density lipoprotein (VLDL) *58*,
    59
vestibulocochlear nerve *62*, 63
Vibrio *74*, 75
villi *22*, 23, *48*, 49
  subtotal atrophy 81
VIPomas 43, 57, *64*, 65
Virchow's node 87
viruses *46*, 47
visceral sensation 45
vitamin(s) *52*, 53
vitamin A *52*, 53
vitamin B-complex *52*, 53
vitamin B deficiencies 13, 17
vitamin B12 33, 49
  absorption *48*, 49, *102*, 103
  coeliac disease 81
  deficiency 53, 55
  digestion *52*, 53
  terminal ileitis 79

vitamin C *52*, 53
  coeliac disease 81
vitamin D *52*, 53
  deficiency 55
  malabsorption 81
vitamin E *52*, 53
vitamin K 49
  coagulation *58*, 59
  digestion *52*, 53
volvulus 101
vomiting 19, 21, *62*, 63
  control 45
  with diarrhoea 65
  dysmotility 41
  gastroenteritis *74*, 75
  pancreatitis 91
  small intestine obstruction 33
  treatment *62*, 63
vomiting centre 35, *62*, 63

warts, peri-anal 39, 89
wasting in cirrhosis *94*, 95
water reabsorption *36*, 37
weight control 55
weight loss 21, 23, 25, 29
  cirrhosis 95
  coeliac disease 81
  small intestinal disorders 33
Werner Morrison syndrome 43
Wernicke's encephalopathy 83
Whipple's disease *76*, 77, 81
Whipple's operation 87
Wilson's disease 29, 53, 61, 94
worms, intestinal 33, *76*, 77

X-rays, plain *100*, 101
xerostomia 15, 17
xylose excretion test *102*, 103

Yersinia enterocolitica 33
Yersinia infection *76*, 77

Z-line *18*, 19
zinc 53
Zollinger–Ellison syndrome 21, 25, 43, 87
  zymogen granules *24*, 25